The Complete Idiot's Reference Card

T'ai Chi is about breathing and relaxing as we move through the changes of life, continually filling and flowing with life energy. By filling with Qi, we become, like Qi, nurturing to all things.

If you remember to breathe, everything else will take care of itself.

Why Am I Doing T'ai Chi?

1. It feels good.
2. It boosts my immune system.
3. It dumps old stress, cleaning my nervous system.
4. It helps me to let go of new stress faster.
5. It makes me more creative and productive.
6. It makes me nicer to be around.
7. It is the best balance and coordination training in the world.
8. It slows my aging process.
9. It keeps me loose and supple, no matter how old I am.
10. It helps process and release "dis-ease" before it becomes a disease.
11. *T'ai Chi improves everything I do!*

T'ai Chi's Philosophy of Living

T'ai Chi means "supreme ultimate." By practicing T'ai Chi, our mind centers, and we become the supreme ultimate point in the universe—a clearer, lighted point from which all that we will ever dream and achieve flows. You become an absolute point of healing, healing yourself, and by so doing, healing the world around you. T'ai Chi celebrates being alive. Daily practice of T'ai Chi's forms cleanses your body and mind of stress, awakens your senses, and opens you to the limitless energy of life—*Qi*.

T'ai Chi gives you an edge, no matter what it is you strive to succeed in. Mor-eover, T'ai Chi teaches us to be happy, excited, and thankful for everything that we are *right now*. This is a wonderful way to live, being here and now, to savor the tremendously exquisite lives we've been given; content and yet ready, willing, and able to take on the noblest adventures in life.

Remember that you are a miracle. You are here to do miraculous things. Sometimes that miraculous thing is just being kind. Enjoy this life; it's the best game in town. Play T'ai Chi, breathe, and everything else will take care of itself.

alpha
books

A T'ai Chi Checklist for Living

➤ Breathe deep, full abdominal breaths whenever you think about it.

➤ Enjoy the passive observation of nature, the sun, or rain.

➤ Really feel the things you touch, the sounds you hear, and really experience the tastes, smells, and sights. *Be here and now each moment.*

➤ Forgive quickly. As T'ai Chi empties the body of held tension, allow the mind and heart to release the past, thereby flowing easily into the future.

➤ Celebrate the pleasure of movement each day as you revel in your T'ai Chi practice, and let that savoring of life weave out into every single thing you do.

T'ai Chi Health Tips

➤ Practice T'ai Chi movements each day.

➤ Practice a deep session of Sitting QiGong each day.

➤ Turn on your Qi, or light energy, anytime you catch yourself being bored.

➤ When obsessive need or anxiety leads you to want unhealthful foods, drinks, or activities, turn on your light energy.

➤ When arguments get out of hand at home or work, walk away and do QiGong or T'ai Chi, before attempting to resolve them.

➤ Before every meeting, interview, test, or any other activity of consequence in your life, do a Sitting QiGong session first. It will help bring all your power into the activity.

➤ Remember that Qi flows effortlessly through you. You do not have to make Qi flow, you only need to let your fears and tensions get out of the way. Qi just happens.

➤ When Qi is flowing, *every* day is a holiday.

Comments on The Complete Idiot's Guide to T'ai Chi & QiGong

I had the privilege of studying T'ai Chi with this book's author, Bill Douglas. As a practicing physician, there are certainly times where stress can seem to be the norm. I found T'ai Chi to be profoundly beneficial in reducing stress, increasing mental clarity, and improving my emotional as well as physical health. Where else can you find such a highly effective tool to achieve these worthwhile goals without fancy equipment or complicated formulas?

I was an emergency room physician when I began studying T'ai Chi with Bill. My first indication of T'ai Chi's powerful stress management benefits came from the ER nurses I worked with, who remarked on my level of serenity during crisis.

If T'ai Chi can help with stress in an ER room where lives often hang in the balance, imagine what it can do for everyone else!

John D.Hernandez, M.D.
Integrative Medicine

Because of my practice of T'ai Chi and QiGong, my barometer for detecting "dis-ease" within myself earlier, allows me to prevent serious infection and speed up healing. I feel T'ai Chi is a wonderful part of a revolution in health care, whereby each of us takes much more responsibility for our own health and healing.

This book can introduce people to the rich esoteric science of T'ai Chi's mind/body fitness in a humorous, easy, and fun way. Enjoy!

Susan Norman, C.I.M.T.

From the perspective of a health psychologist serving patients who are coping with chronic illness and stressful life events, I see the gentle mindfulness exercises of T'ai Chi and QiGong relaxation therapy as potentially useful for a broad spectrum of people. The author of this book, Bill Douglas, explains the complexities of T'ai Chi and QiGong in the form of an invitation, easing his students into a greater understanding of the usefulness and purpose of this ancient form of meditative movement.

Kristy Straits-Troster, Ph.D., Clinical Psychologist, Primary Care Medicine

Dizziness is one of the more common reasons for a doctor visit, particularly in patients over the age of fifty. Because the causes of dizziness can range from benign self-limiting conditions to potentially life threatening ones, a thorough medical evaluation is essential before embarking on any form of therapy. Persistent dizziness certainly has a distinct impact on the quality of life and emotional well being of the patient. Falls, hip fractures and lack of confidence in public often create a feeling of helplessness.

In over twenty years of experience as a clinical neurologist, I find that extensive and expensive medical evaluation including CAT scans, MRI scans and vascular imaging studies as well as prescription medications add little to alleviating the problem. I have found vestibular rehabilitation exercises in the form of T'ai Chi classes to be a cost-effective mode of therapy. Many of my patients have opted for this non-medication approach to treatment and have developed a sense of self-confidence through this form of exercise. In short, as a traditional medical practitioner, I frequently recommend T'ai Chi for my patients with dizziness and dysequilibrium.

Charles D. Donohoe, M.D.
Neurologist

It has been a year since I began practicing T'ai Chi under the teaching of the author of this book, Bill Douglas and his associate instructor Erik Feagans. This span of time certainly allows me to evaluate the result of this gentle "martial art," not only as stress management therapy but, more impressively, with regard to its effect on my physical health.

Suffering for years from chronic neck pain consequent to a whiplash injury, and also suffering from a limited motion of the right shoulder, I approached the T'ai Chi course with some skepticism. The course was initiated after unsuccessful sessions of physical therapy, including mobilization, ultrasounds, heat application, etc. After two months of T'ai Chi, the pain in the cervical region disappeared while the range of motion of my right shoulder returned completely to normal. This achievement remained unchanged during the past winter up until now.

I would not hesitate to recommend T'ai Chi to individuals suffering from the same ailments as well as to mature persons who are seeking to maintain or improve their health and to remain free of chronic pain due to the aging process.

Loredana Brizio-Molteni, M.D., F.A.C.S.

I have been, since many years, interested in the oriental arts and philosophy, including the "martial arts." It took however my wife's persistence to persuade me to enlist in your T'ai Chi courses, which I have been taking since July 1997.

My attitude, since the first few lessons, changed, due to your effectiveness and to your ability to teach this gentle "martial art." I was suffering for symptoms related to osteoarthritis of the left coxofemoral joint, and, in addition, I was suffering from neck pain with limited motion. This symptomology disappeared with the T'ai Chi exercises.

My physician's recommendation is to continue with the practice of T'ai Chi. I would pass the same recommendation to individuals with similar sedentary life styles as well as to people involved in activity, which requires exertion of the musculo-skeletal system.

Agostino Molteni, M.D., Ph.D.

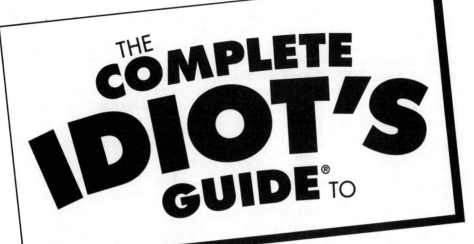

THE COMPLETE IDIOT'S GUIDE® TO

T'ai Chi & QiGong

by Bill Douglas

alpha books

A Division of Macmillan General Reference
An Ahsuog, Inc. Company
1633 Broadway, New York, NY 10019-6785

Macmillan Publishing books may be purchased for business or sales promotional use. For information please write: Special Markets Department, Macmillan Publishing USA, 1633 Broadway, New York, NY 10019.

International Standard Book Number: 0-02-862909-4
Library of Congress Catalog Card Number: 98-85971

01 00 99   8 7 6 5 4 3 2

Interpretation of the printing code: the rightmost number of the first series of numbers is the year of the book's printing; the rightmost number of the second series of numbers is the number of the book's printing. For example, a printing code of 99-1 shows that the first printing occurred in 1999.

Printed in the United States of America

Alpha Development Team

Publisher
Kathy Nebenhaus

Editorial Director
Gary M. Krebs

Managing Editor
Bob Shuman

Marketing Brand Manager
Felice Primeau

Development Editors
Phil Kitchel
Al McDermid
Amy Zavatto

Production Team

Production Editor
Mark Enochs

Copy Editor
Cliff Shubbs

Cover Designer
Mike Freeland

Photo Editor
Richard H. Fox

Illustrator
Jody P. Schaeffer

Designer
Nathan Clement

Indexer
Chris Wilcox

Layout/Proofreading
Melissa Auciello-Brogan
Carrie Allen
Jerry Cole
Laura Goetz
Angel Perez

Contents at a Glance

Contents

Foreword

As Bill explains in this book, although T'ai Chi and Qigong are exercises, they are integral parts of Traditional Chinese Medicine (TCM). As alternative medicine and therapies sweep the Western world, doctors now prescribe QiGong and T'ai Chi for treating stress problems, illnesses, and injuries, while many people use it as a tonic to extend their peak performance into old age. Robert Parish, one of the great NBA players claimed T'ai Chi extended his career, making him one of the oldest *dominant* starting players in NBA history. Just as T'ai Chi protected Mr. Parish's body from the intense stress of professional basketball, it can help each of us protect ourselves from the relentless stress of a rapidly changing world.

In my 43 years of experience in Traditional Chinese Medicine, here and in the Orient, I have never heard anyone explain the premise of T'ai Chi and QiGong as succinctly as Bill does. He has the most unusual ability to explain concepts he's spent a lifetime learning in a way that is tangible and applicable to the novice student the very first day of class. You will happily realize this book offers you, the reader, a humorous and enjoyable journey deep into the world of T'ai Chi and QiGong. After providing an extensive understanding of T'ai Chi and QiGong's profound potential, the book proceeds to very practically explain how you can dive into T'ai Chi and QiGong by clarifying such basic concepts as what to wear to class and what to call your teacher.

This book provides ways T'ai Chi can be integrated into your life on many levels through your work, social-recreation, and healthcare, just as it has been in China for many years. Bill shares and eloquently articulates my vision that Traditional Chinese Medicine is leading a transformation in Western health-care that will financially save you, the patient, untold dollars and much needless pain and suffering. This book will facilitate that transformation by making the everyday person comfortable with the common sense approach health tools like T'ai Chi and QiGong make, and we will all be better for it.

This book, with humor and gentleness, guides you through T'ai Chi and QiGong to help you boost your immune system, sleep better, and improve everything about you effortlessly. This book is for everybody living with stress, but a must for every corporate wellness director, healthcare worker, and activities director. Here you can learn why T'ai Chi is the fastest growing exercise and healing balm for modern life!

—**Richard Yennie**, D.C., Dipl. Ac. (NCCA)

Deputy Director, China Medical Assn., Research Committee, Taipei, Taiwan; President, QiGong Society of America; U.S. Representative, World Academic Society of Medical QiGong; President, Acupuncture Society of America, Inc.; Faculty Member, Waseda Acupuncture College, Tokyo, Japan; Visiting Professor at Beijing University of Chinese Medicine, Beijing, China; Dean of Academic Affairs, Kansas College of Chinese Medicine, Wichita, KS; Winner of Doctor of the Year Award for outstanding achievement in TCM by the Sixth International Congress of Chinese Medicine, First Place USA, and Second Place International Award.

How to Use This Book

This book is divided into six parts. Each part's information will prepare you for the next, opening your mind and imagination to concepts that will unlock your ability to expand your awareness of T'ai Chi and QiGong even more.

Part 1, "T'ai Chi: Relax into It," explains how T'ai Chi and QiGong can change every part of your life for the better. Part 1 concludes in explaining how T'ai Chi and QiGong work by introducing you to Traditional Chinese Medicine and explaining how modern Western science is now beginning to understand how this ancient wisdom works.

Part 2, "Suiting Up and Setting Out," will prepare you to dive into T'ai Chi and QiGong "big time" or "little time," depending on how much of T'ai Chi's magic you want to experience. Here you will learn the nuts and bolts of how classes are taught, T'ai Chi etiquette, terms, wardrobe, and all the things that will enable you to choose the best class for you.

However, Part 2 will also explain the underlying tenets of T'ai Chi and QiGong. Not only will you look knowledgeable and informed to others on the outside, but you will be able to assimilate the deep and profound benefits of T'ai Chi and QiGong much quicker and more effectively. Whether you learn T'ai Chi from a live class or a video-tape, these chapters will greatly enhance your experience. In fact, even experienced T'ai Chi practitioners can benefit from this section's insights.

Part 3, "Starting Down the QiGong Path to T'ai Chi," explains how QiGong works and then leads you into an experience that is exquisite beyond words. This part ends with an introduction to Moving QiGong exercises that include the warm ups that prepare your mind and body to dive into an ocean of T'ai Chi experience. T'ai Chi literally means "the supreme ultimate," so hold on for an incredible ride!

Part 4, "Kuang Ping T'ai Chi: Walk on Life's Lighter Side," illuminates the history of T'ai Chi and how the Kuang Ping Yang Style was brought to the West by Master Kuo Lien Ying. Then you will be led through the entire 64 postures of this powerful ancient form and instructed as to a few of the benefits of each movement. Yet, remember the benefits are endless, and since this book is only about 300 pages long, to discover them you must experience them yourself as they unfold beautifully within you every day for the rest of your life.

Part 5, "T'ai Chi's Buffet of Short, Sword and Fan Styles," exposes you to the many incredibly beautiful forms of T'ai Chi that are available to you today. Remember that only about 30 years ago, these arts were secrets of China, so we are very lucky to have these exquisite art forms available to us now in our lifetimes. Part 5 will give you a small, yet delicious, taste of what is available. If you seek, ye shall find.

Part 6, "Life Applications," shows that T'ai Chi is much more than just a "physical exercise." T'ai Chi can help heal every aspect of our lives, our relationships, and our world. Part 6 will explain how T'ai Chi and/or QiGong can be used to help treat almost any illness or physical malady and how T'ai Chi can be a powerful adjunct therapy for many mental or emotional problems as well. T'ai Chi's philosophy of life can improve your diet and life skills, as well, by teaching you about the balance of yin and yang forces.

Lastly, Part 6 will give you all the ammo you need to get your company to invest in T'ai Chi classes and T'ai Chi breaks for you and your coworkers. Part 6 will not only give you information on why T'ai Chi should also be a part of our education, healthcare, senior service programs, and most other aspects of the community, but will give you ideas on how to make this happen.

T'ai Chi Pearls

Throughout this book, we'll be adding five types of extra information in boxes, for your enlightenment:

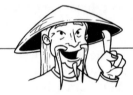

Sage Sifu Says

Sage Sifu Says boxes will offer you tips on living the principles of T'ai Chi and will maximize your understanding of T'ai Chi's subtle layers to help you get the most out of it. Sifu (pronounced *see-foo*) means "one who has mastered an art." Not only martial arts, but a master chef, or artist, might be a sifu.

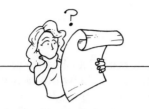

Know Your Chinese

These boxes will give you definitions for Chinese medical and philosophical terms related to T'ai Chi and QiGong. Pronunciations are given as well.

T'ai Sci

T'ai Chi Science boxes provide you modern scientific terms and insights into the world of T'ai Chi's ancient discoveries.

Ouch!

These boxes will alert you to any caution you should observe in T'ai Chi practice. There won't be many of these. T'ai Chi injuries are nearly nonexistent when done correctly.

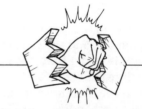

A T'ai Chi Punch Line

T'ai Chi Punch Line boxes are full of fun anecdotes and trivia about the fascinating world of T'ai Chi and QiGong, modern and old.

Acknowledgements

A great thanks to the many dedicated Chinese creators of T'ai Chi who've spent lifetimes developing this wonderful art and health science the world now has access to. T'ai Chi and QiGong are great gifts the Chinese culture has provided for the world, and I offer them a deep and heartfelt thank you. Their efforts leave me convinced that every culture on this planet has treasures to offer the rest, and I hope we all can open our hearts and minds to truth and value no matter where it comes from.

A profound thanks to my teacher, Master Jennifer Booth, her teacher Gil Messenger, their teacher Russell Schofield, and our grand master Kuo Lien Ying, who made the daunting journey from China to San Francisco. His courage in migrating to this strange land made it possible for millions of Americans to have access to the beauty and power of Kuang Ping Yang T'ai Chi Chuan.

I would like to thank my brilliant sister Diane Douglas, her associates Jay and Sandra, my brother Ed, and sisters Barbara and Peggy, without whose insights and support, none of this would have been possible. My wife Angela and her mother Shun Oi Wong were an integral part of my T'ai Chi journey, and my father-in-law, Bonwyn Wong, embodied the humility and infinite wisdom Chinese people are famous for. My children Isaac, Andrea, and Michael led me to the doorway of change through their innocent examples of wisdom, and my parents, Evelyn and William Douglas, showed me that even the harshest tests can produce pearls in we beautiful creatures known as human beings.

Thanks to Mulan Quan instructors Angela Wong-Douglas and Andrea Mei-Wah Douglas for their wonderful exhibitions and insights into the elegant art form of Mulan Quan basic, fan and sword style. Thanks to my superb agent Debra Rodman, editors Gary Krebs and Al McDermid, and for Susan Norman's sage advice on holistic living.

Thanks to my students and assistant instructors Erik, Liz, Dan, Denny, Twila, Allen, Karl, Nan, Linda, Sari, Bill, Hallee, Nancy, Janet, Joel, Diane, Sharon, and everyone I've failed to mention for enabling me to expand my understanding of T'ai Chi by teaching it to them.

Special thanks to Heather Boyle, A Visionary in Corporate Wellness Consulting, and for my friend Jeff Chappell's support.

David Larson (photos) e-mail: davidlarson@sprintmail.com

Jenny Hahn (sketch artist) e-mail: shikuns@gvi.net

Jessica Kincaid (computer graphics): www.filigree.com

Part 1
T'ai Chi: Relax into It!

Part 1 explains why a simple, easy-to-do, 2,000-year-old Chinese martial art is the most popular exercise in the world today and is practiced in corporations, hospitals, living rooms, and backyards (just like yours) around the world.

If you want to find a calm center in the middle of life's storm of change, while also toning your muscles and healing your mind and body, T'ai Chi and QiGong are just what the doctor ordered (literally, ask your doctor!).

T'ai Chi is a unique exercise that simultaneously heals the physical, mental, emotional, and spiritual body. With T'ai Chi, you can boost your energy levels, dramatically improve your health, slow your aging process, become more creative, and significantly lower your stress levels even in our increasingly stressful world. And this is only scratching the surface of T'ai Chi's benefits.

Part 1 will show you that all the power you ever needed is found right in the center of where you are anytime and all the time. Providing access to the unlimited personal power that we each possess makes T'ai Chi perhaps the most powerful personal growth tool in the world. So, whether you seek a simple, easy-to-do exercise, a stress-management tool, or a profoundly healthy philosophy of life, T'ai Chi may just be what you've been looking for.

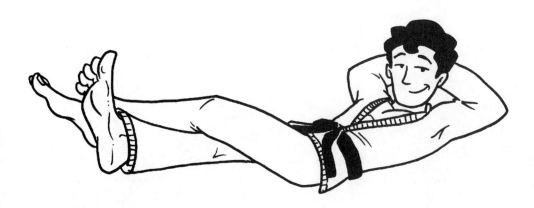

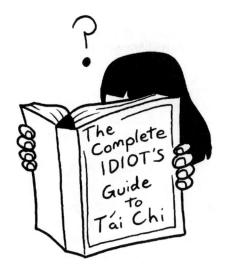

Chapter 1

Why Practice T'ai Chi?

In This Chapter

➤ Why is T'ai Chi so popular?

➤ What T'ai Chi can do for you

➤ Is T'ai Chi a fountain of youth?

➤ T'ai Chi is exercise with much gain and no pain

➤ T'ai Chi teaches self acceptance

T'ai Chi is practiced by 20 percent of the world's population and is fast becoming the most popular exercise in the world today. Its rapid expansion is largely due to one important fact—*it feels really good*. Although T'ai Chi was originally a martial art and is increasingly offered by martial arts studios, it's now practiced in businesses, hospitals, and schools everywhere. T'ai Chi is not only a valuable tool for improving health, it is a powerful business tool as well. Companies see that T'ai Chi improves productivity by helping employees to be happy, relaxed, and creative. Hospitals see T'ai Chi as a potent, yet cost-effective, therapy for nearly any condition. T'ai Chi classes can be found nowadays almost anywhere.

Do you ever feel like life is getting more stressful? *It is*. The increasing stress in today's world is one reason for T'ai Chi's growing worldwide popularity. T'ai Chi was designed to help people go through change with less damage by improving the way we handle stress. Studies show change is stressful, and *even though change is often good*, if the stress that change causes isn't managed it can damage our health and outlook on life. Since about 90 percent of the discoveries made in the history of the human race have been made in our lifetime, we are all going through some serious change—*and stress*. Therefore, T'ai Chi's ability to help practitioners "let go" of this stress more easily is just what the doctor ordered, *literally*.

Imagine life is a carousel upon which we ride. When life gets spinning really fast, T'ai Chi seems to slow things down, like a hand pulling us away from the "edge," back to the center of life's carousel. Here, *in the center*, we can let life spin even faster and not feel like throwing up (*hardly ever anyway*). In fact, by practicing T'ai Chi as you ride life's carousel, you might even catch yourself going "wheeeeeeeeeeeeee" a lot more often.

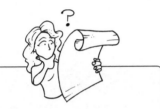

Know Your Chinese

The Chinese call life energy **Qi** (pronounced *chee*). The character for Qi is also the character for air or breath. QiGong (pronounced *chee kung* and often spelled Chi–Gong) means "breath work" or "energy exercise." There are about 7,000 QiGong exercises in the Chinese Medica (the bible of Chinese Medicine). T'ai Chi is a moving form of QiGong. There are sitting and lying forms of QiGong, but all T'ai Chi is done standing and moving.

Whether you are stressed out, continually exhausted, treating a health problem, or just wanting to get in shape and feel young again, T'ai Chi is just what you need. T'ai Chi goes right to the heart of everything we do by healing and cleansing the central nervous system. T'ai Chi helps us to let go of all the nervous tension that bogs down our mental computer system (like getting a general tune up every day). This makes everything inside us work better, which often makes the world around us seem better, too. So T'ai Chi is really a self-improvement tool that will make you a better "anything-you-want-to-be." Unless of course you want to be stressed out, exhausted, uninspired, and feel old and out of shape. In that case, T'ai Chi won't help.

People everywhere in the world are rapidly embracing T'ai Chi as "their" exercise. Although T'ai Chi originates from China, it is now seen so commonly in the West that soon it will be thought of as an American thing, a British thing, a Canadian thing, or whatever. If you ask American kids what their favorite American food is, many will reply, "PIZZA!" (which is originally Italian). And someday, when asked what their favorite American pastime is, Americans will say, "T'AI CHI!"

How T'ai Chi Works

Just as we flow through the changes of life (or not), our life energy, or *Qi*, flows through us (or not, if we are stressed out). Qi is the energy of life and flows through all living things. Qi animates, heals, and nurtures life. When the stress of change makes us tense, we squeeze off the flow of life energy. Physically, this feels like tension. T'ai Chi and QiGong are easy, simple, yet sophisticated relaxation exercises that encourage the muscles to let go of tension, the mind to let go of worry, and the heart to let go of angst. Tension, worry, and angst all block our Qi flow.

Tension, worry, and angst are usually the result of our mind, heart, or body being unable to "let go" of something. The goal of T'ai Chi is to move through a series of choreographed movements like a slow martial arts routine, but *very* slowly and in a state of absolute relaxation. In order to do this, we have to let go of our mental/physical tensions, grudges, prejudices, and anything that keeps us tied to the past. This enables us to flow more easily into the future by clearing our mind and body of old stress so that we constantly get a "fresh" perspective on life.

T'ai Chi is simple and easy to do, yet benefits us on many deep and complex levels. T'ai Chi's slow, relaxed movements incorporate breathing and relaxation techniques that cleanse our mind, body, and emotions each time we go through the gentle movements. T'ai Chi is designed to uncover and release every single place we hold tension or blocked energy. When our mind or heart holds onto issues (fears, obsession, angers, and so on) our body literally squeezes itself with tension. Going slowly through the movements is like doing an internal scan of the entire body to clear and release any place the body is gripping onto tension. There is no exercise on earth that can help you go through this wild ride toward the future quite like T'ai Chi can—which is why T'ai Chi is truly the exercise of the future.

Is T'ai Chi a Martial Art?

T'ai Chi looks very much like slow motion kung fu. David Carradine performed T'ai Chi as Kwai Chang Cane on the television series *Kung Fu*. And although T'ai Chi shares some similarities with kung fu, don't let that scare you away. T'ai Chi can be practiced by anyone at any age and in any condition.

In martial arts circles, it is known as an internal martial art. T'ai Chi promotes internal strength physically, mentally, and emotionally, which is why it can be powerful training tool for martial artists. But you don't have to be a martial artist to benefit from T'ai Chi because it can also be practiced even by those in wheelchairs, with great results.

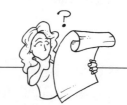

Know Your Chinese

T'ai Chi Ch'uan (pronounced *tie chee chwan* or *die gee jwan*), sometimes spelled Taijiquan, means "supreme ultimate fist," or "highest martial art." T'ai means Supreme. Chi means Ultimate. Ch'uan means Fist.

How Do You Measure T'ai Chi Progress?

Unlike karate, T'ai Chi has no belt or ranking system because the benefits of T'ai Chi can only be *felt* and not seen. You practice T'ai Chi to live better, more calmly, clearly, healthfully, and productively. T'ai Chi is a tonic for life. You will see your progress reflected by how you feel, how spry you look in the mirror, how much you love life, and how healthy you are. Isn't this much better than owning a black belt? However, if you do karate, T'ai Chi can help you get that black belt by improving your internal function and grace.

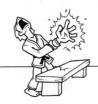

Ouch

Nearly 1/3 of the adult U.S. population has chronic high blood pressure. Since some medications have side effects, physicians need to be made aware that T'ai Chi can sometimes lower high blood pressure as effectively as medication. Ask your doctor to look into T'ai Chi. However, never adjust medication levels without consulting your physician.

Everybody Is Doing It!

Also, T'ai Chi differs from most martial arts in that people of all ages can practice it. Many people with disabilities and ailments practice T'ai Chi as therapy. No one is restricted from practicing T'ai Chi, and yet T'ai Chi can benefit the fittest athletes, just as much as it benefits elderly arthritis sufferers. T'ai Chi clubs are sprouting up all over the world, with people from all walks of life.

Going to the Root of Problems

Life is very complicated, and T'ai Chi cannot solve all your problems. However, T'ai Chi can help you simplify your life in a big and relaxing way.

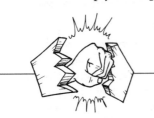

A T'ai Chi Punch Line

One old Chinese master lecturing his new students said, "QiGong is said to build character in its practitioners. I don't know about that, but it will definitely make you into a character."

Imagine that you're a tree. While your mind and body are the trunk of that tree, all your "life stuff" is like the many leaves on that tree. Your job, relationships, hobbies, hopes, and problems are all dangling out there on the tips of your life. When your health is bad or you can't sleep well, this affects the whole tree. You may have problems with your job that may strain your relationships, which in turn will drain the energy you need to pursue your hobbies, making you too tired to have hopeful dreams, *and causing your problems to get seemingly bigger and bigger*. When you are already beat, trying to figure out how to heal all these sick, shriveled leaves is too much to even think about.

However, what if you could pour some magic water on the roots of your tree? Magic that would heal all the sick

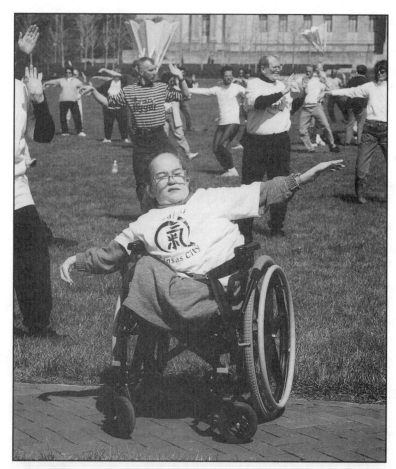

T'ai Chi is increasingly popular!

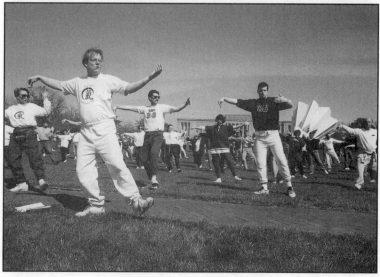

Bill Douglas (yes, the author of this book) leads the Kansas City T'ai Chi Club in the largest gathering of T'ai Chi practitioners outside China.

leaves and cause them to grow larger, to catch more breezes and more sunlight, *and more fun!* This is what T'ai Chi does. By nurturing the very core of our mind and body, T'ai Chi makes us better at *everything we do*. We don't practice T'ai Chi to be better at T'ai Chi (although that happens). Each time we practice T'ai Chi, we pour healing water on the roots of everything we are. This healing water, or energy, is carried out to the leaves of everything we do, making us the freshest, greenest tree we could ever want to be.

Getting to the Root of T'ai Chi

One name does not adequately express everything T'ai Chi is because T'ai Chi nurtures so many aspects of our lives at the root. Although originally a martial art known as T'ai Chi Chuan ("supreme ultimate fist"), the shortened name of *T'ai Chi* reflects how it is now viewed, as one of the most effective mind/body exercise in the world. So, T'ai Chi now refers to "supreme ultimate health exercise," "supreme ultimate relaxation therapy," "supreme ultimate balance conditioner, muscle toner, beauty treatment."

T'ai Chi is the supreme ultimate because it goes right to the root of most health problems by relaxing the muscles and mind, aligning the spinal posture, and balancing the energy systems that run through the body, providing them with life energy. It is one of the most soothing, easy, and powerful things you can do for yourself. It is a profound self-improvement tool, a great toning exercise, and an incredible healing art.

T'ai Chi Root Benefits; Let Me Count the Ways...

T'ai Chi is an all-purpose therapy, and millions around the world practice it for many different reasons. Whether you want to improve external beauty, mental outlook, or physical health and longevity, T'ai Chi heals the roots of your being.

All-Purpose Medicine

T'ai Chi is a highly effective therapy for many injuries or chronic conditions, whether mental, emotional, or physical. The following chapters will discuss different maladies and how T'ai Chi treats them. T'ai Chi bolsters the immune system, as well, and can actually eliminate problems long before they become an actual physical illness.

An Ultimate Beauty Treatment

Forget about covering up problems with makeup or surgery. Beautify from the inside out instead! Many cells are replaced daily, and almost the entire body is completely replaced every five to seven years. We are literally born anew on some level each and every day of our lives. How those cells are reproduced is determined by how the life energy, or Qi, flows through our body. Therefore, we can have a terrific impact on how we age, look, and feel by promoting our Qi flow.

T'ai Chi Power: T'ai Chi Washes the Nervous System

Have you ever sat back and noticed how small children never run down? Like the Energizer rabbit, on fast forward, they leap and spring, dance and chat, and chat and chat. Have you ever thought to yourself, "God, I wish *I* had that energy?" Well, you *do* have access to that energy (and without doing espresso shooters).

We begin to block our access to that energy as we "mature" by holding onto past grudges, by shouldering responsibilities that are unrealistic, or just because of silly worries. Then we don't know how to let them go, and we get used to having less and less energy. We can think on a mental level that we want to "stop worrying" or "let go of tension," but that doesn't really work. We need life tools that help us let go of these blocks on deep levels in our mind, heart, and body, so that we can open to our flow of life energy.

T'ai Chi and QiGong will give you access to simple exercises, which feel good and can open a valve to that limitless energy you thought you had lost forever. The Chinese discovered long ago that these blocks, or our stress, are simply the mind and nervous system squeezing onto grudges, worries, or even desires. Just as our muscles can tighten when tense, our mind and heart can grip

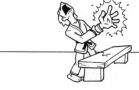

Ouch

T'ai Chi can boost your energy levels tremendously. However, it is important also to get the proper amount of sleep. Do not try to use T'ai Chi's energy boost to replace proper sleep and diet. T'ai Chi will promote an all-around healthful lifestyle as you become more subtly attuned to your body's needs. One aspect of T'ai Chi's quiet mindful movement is that it quiets us down enough to sense the mind and body's needs, whether it's more rest, water, and so on.

tension too, and we have to be taught how to let go of their squeezing grip on life issues. So, the goal of these ancient exercises is to wash our nervous system clean, so our mind can be fresh and vibrant like a newborn baby's, while still remembering the important stuff, like stopping at red lights and dressing before going to work.

Seriously, as we let go of most of the meaningless, irritating debris bouncing around in our mind, we have more space and energy for really important ideas to surface. Important memories like the bill you forgot to pay, or realizations like the person you forgot to tell that you care about them. T'ai Chi's slow, soothing movements provide that calm open space, even in the very center of the rat race.

The Fountain of Youth!

America is not into the "aging" thing. What we spend on cosmetic surgery attests to that. T'ai Chi will help you get over that prejudice, while also slowing the aging process in many ways. The Chinese believe T'ai Chi will return us to a state of "child-likeness" (but not childishness), where we see the world with fresh eyes. This allows us the freedom to reinvent ourselves easily and constantly, *just as children do*, enabling us to flow with the changes of life. We can once again be flexible and exuberant, while still benefiting from the wisdom of experience (like being able to hit our mouth with the spoon, well, most of the time). So, T'ai Chi has the ability to renew us, and through that renewal enhance our strength, health, and creativity.

T'ai Chi is based on the principle that the world doesn't need to be held up by our worrying mind and tense body. In fact, we are much more helpful to the world (and far more enjoyable to be around) if we can let go of as much stress as possible. Realizing this principle is the first big step to letting T'ai Chi reopen you to your own personal rejuvenating "fountain of energy"!

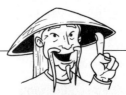

Sage Sifu Says

I used to hold the world on my shoulders
'til my tense muscles felt like very heavy boulders.
Then one day Sifu said, "This world needs no holders,
so breathe and relax your bony little shoulders."
...so I did!

A T'ai Chi Poem

No More "Drop and Give Me Twenty!"

T'ai Chi is popular because it is easy to do and provides a gentle workout that doesn't leave you drained, *but energized!* T'ai Chi's "effortless" nature is a big stretch for most of us, however, because we associate exercise with *force*, *pain*, and *tension*. In fact, some exercise actually contributes to stress. When I played junior high football in west Texas many years ago, the coaches determined that we were through running when one of us started throwing up. That's right, upchucking. It was the only time in my life I ever hoped to see someone throw up.

T'ai Chi Is an Exercise That Feels Good

T'ai Chi is helping the world get a healthy, enjoyable view of exercise. As a nation, we have adopted a mutant notion of exercise, exemplified by the mantra "no pain, no gain." This has traumatized many Americans, including myself, leaving an indelible mark on how we view exercise. In T'ai Chi we have a mantra too, "If your exercise causes pain, you'll get so sick of the thought of it that you'll never want to do it again." Ours isn't as neatly poetic as "no pain, no gain," but ours makes infinitely more sense. T'ai Chi should always, always, *always,* feel good. And since it does feel good, you will look forward to it. Each morning you will find yourself grateful that you're alive and able to practice this cool exercise called T'ai Chi.

You Are Perfect and Perfect for T'ai Chi

T'ai Chi's accepting nature makes it very popular. Everyone is *qualified* to do T'ai Chi. You don't have to look good in tights or Spandex to do T'ai Chi, although if you do T'ai Chi enough, you'll look pretty good in whatever you like to wear.

T'ai Chi and QiGong are for anybody who is dealing with stress. In other words—*everybody*. Anybody can do T'ai Chi, including people in wheelchairs. If you've picked up a book on T'ai Chi, you've probably experienced the *acute stress* of imagining yourself in some of those incredible (seemingly impossible) positions the T'ai Chi models pose in for the photos. Relax. Those people are models. Most people do T'ai Chi just the way you will do it. Easily and effortlessly. Although T'ai Chi was one of the original martial arts, it is now practiced all over the world as a relaxation technique by people of all ages in the same shape you are in, and sometimes *in even worse shape.*

When we begin an exercise class, we have the illusion that everybody other than us "belongs" there, and that they are all "good" at it. You will find that everybody goes through the same trials and tribulations. As you lighten up on yourself, you'll see struggling, growing, and healing are everywhere. Breathe and enjoy; you are among friends.

Explaining T'ai Chi: History and Premise

T'ai Chi is unique. Although it is in a way 2,000 years old, it is at the cutting edge of modern Western medical research. T'ai Chi is ancient yet modern, Eastern yet increasingly Western. Using

Ouch

Beginning T'ai Chi is a *big step* for many of us, and it is easy to psych yourself out of taking it. Just like the first day we went to kindergarten, we thought of all the "big bad" stuff that would probably happen. But, for most of us, none of that materialized, and in fact we actually had a lot of fun. Take a chance. Dive into life by entering the waters of T'ai Chi and QiGong.

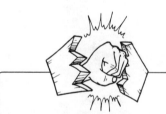

A T'ai Chi Punch Line

When you first begin practicing T'ai Chi out in the backyard or in your local park, people may stare. Before long, your unique practice of T'ai Chi becomes part of the rich texture of the neighborhood, and if you move away, they will miss you. Just as T'ai Chi adds to your personal internal charm, your practice adds to the charm of your community.

11

T'ai Sci

Western science is embracing T'ai Chi very rapidly. Almost every month a new study seems to find yet another thing T'ai Chi can treat, cure, or improve. T'ai Chi is rapidly becoming a part of modern Western medicine and modern life.

T'ai Chi is a way to get the most benefit out of all worlds, old and new, East and West.

Have you ever been pulled over for moving too slowly? You've got some T'ai Chi explaining to do. One of my students was practicing T'ai Chi in the park in a suburb of Kansas City one morning when a patrol car pulled up to ask if he was all right. The officer said someone had called and reported somebody was having a "problem" in the park. So, it may behoove you to know a bit more about T'ai Chi in case you need to do some fast-talking. The following will help.

Historical T'ai Chi

For an exercise that is so made to order for modern life, it is amazing to realize that T'ai Chi is thought to be about 1,200 years old. Furthermore, T'ai Chi is an expanded version of a more ancient exercise called QiGong, which may be at least 2,000 years old. T'ai Chi's moving exercises are done very slowly, like slow motion kung fu. In days of old, T'ai Chi (or T'ai Chi Ch'uan) was primarily a martial art. It is believed that Buddhist and Taoist monks began practicing T'ai Chi forms in monasteries (Yes, like the Shao Lin Temple) for two reasons. One, to promote health because they were out of shape from sitting around meditating all the time. And two, because they were so out of shape, they couldn't defend themselves, and bandits would come and beat them up before taking their valuables. (*And you thought you had stress!*)

T'ai Sci

Biofeedback uses a computer program to train people how to relax when under stress. The computer shows them when their blood pressure goes up and their heart beats faster so that they can then practice relaxing and slowing things down. Dr. Gary Green, a leading biofeedback specialist, refers to T'ai Chi as "biofeedback without the computer."

Modern T'ai Chi

When most people first join a T'ai Chi or QiGong class, they are not quite sure what they are getting themselves into. Most have a mother, a doctor, a friend, a daughter, or son telling them, "This T'ai Chi stuff is the greatest thing since sliced bread and you have gotta' try it!" However, these enthusiasts can't quite explain why you've gotta' try it. So, the following is for you, or whoever's been trying to explain it to you.

In modern terms, T'ai Chi and QiGong are ancient systems of *biofeedback* and classical conditioning. Traditional Chinese doctors of long ago noted that our natural tendency is to hold onto stress, which bogs down the brain. They therefore created exercises that would train the mind and the body not only to continually dump stress, but also to actually change the way the body handles future stress (not the way your kids change the way you handle stress, but *in a good way*).

As T'ai Chi players move through their slow motion movements, their mind becomes calm, their breathing deepens and slows, and their muscles relax. All this happens while the muscles are toning, making it a very efficient exercise. But, forget about efficiency, T'ai Chi should be done as though you were going to do it forever. If you try to "hurry up and relax," it doesn't work as well.

The Least You Need to Know

➤ T'ai Chi reduces stress and slows the aging process.

➤ Everybody can do T'ai Chi.

➤ T'ai Chi restores the power of youthful exuberance.

➤ T'ai Chi is an efficient therapy that can improve all aspects of our lives.

➤ By clearing the mind, T'ai Chi reminds us that life is a miracle.

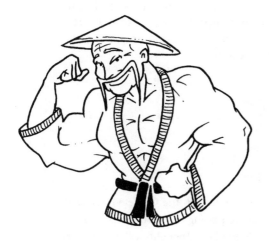

Chapter 2

Let's Get Physical

In This Chapter

➤ T'ai Chi tunes up the whole you

➤ T'ai Chi's an *inner-cise*

➤ Beauty inside *and* out

➤ Losing weight healthfully with T'ai Chi

➤ What is a "dan tien?"

➤ T'ai Chi is the ultimate performance booster

➤ T'ai Chi vs. yoga; both are good so what's the diff?

T'ai Chi is perhaps the best physical exercise in the world. Unlike higher impact exercises, T'ai Chi does not harm the body. In fact, its gentle movements help the body strengthen bone mass and connective tissue, and are lower impact than even brisk walking. T'ai Chi also works on a cellular level to physically cleanse and tone the body in deep ways that you never see. However, T'ai Chi can help beautify the external physical body, too.

Depending on the type of T'ai Chi work out, you may not even break a sweat doing T'ai Chi. Therefore, T'ai Chi is a great workout you can do during a fifteen minute coffee break at work, in your regular work clothes, or in your pajamas when you get up. It won't leave you out of breath and fatigued, but it will leave you feeling clear, peaceful, and at one with the universe.

According to some studies, T'ai Chi burns nearly as many calories as downhill skiing and provides many of the same health benefits as low-impact aerobic exercises. However, T'ai Chi provides balance and coordination improvements that are nearly twice as effective as the best balance training exercises in the world.

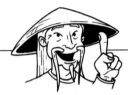

Sage Sifu Says

T'ai Chi provides the most benefits when it is done for fun. In fact, the Chinese refer to T'ai Chi practice as *playing* T'ai Chi. Always remember you are playing (as opposed to "working out"), and play T'ai Chi simply because playing it feels good—the benefits will come easily and naturally. To do T'ai Chi everyday and not get T'ai Chi's multitudinous benefits would be like falling down and missing the ground—you just can't do it.

If you are an athlete, T'ai Chi could also be the best training you can do to improve your game. Golfers sometimes add a hundred yards to their drives after "playing" T'ai Chi for just a few months, while weight lifters often see results immediately. Yet, even if your main physical activity is mowing the lawn and carrying groceries, the same things T'ai Chi does to benefit athletic performance will increase your physical power and dramatically reduce the likelihood of injury when working around the house.

There is no single exercise that can do what T'ai Chi does for you physically. This is why T'ai Chi is becoming the most popular exercise in the world today.

T'ai Sci

Acupuncture stimulates points on the body that affect the flow of Qi, or life energy. Acupressure is acupuncture without the needles. By massaging acupuncture points you are performing acupressure and getting much the same benefit.

T'ai Chi Acupuncture Tune Up

T'ai Chi is a very slow exercise, performed as if you were swimming through water, or the air in T'ai Chi's case. This has many benefits. You cannot injure yourself when doing T'ai Chi correctly because the slowness allows you time to hear the body's pain signals and stop any movement that doesn't feel right. You simply adjust the T'ai Chi movements to fit your own range of mobility.

T'ai Chi's slow standing movements also thoroughly massage the bottoms of the feet. There are acupuncture points on the feet that affect every part of the body, including every major organ. Therefore, the gentle slow massaging of the feet that your 20-minute T'ai Chi routine accomplishes treats the entire body. By the end of your T'ai Chi play time, every cell of the body will be relaxed and opened to a smoother flow of life energy. You will feel clear, bright, and renewed. The science of acupuncture is explained in greater detail later in the book.

Innercise vs. Outercise

T'ai Chi is a mind/body exercise, or an *inner-cise*. That is, T'ai Chi aids the mind and body simultaneously to powerfully center us, to improve not only our physical health, but also our mental and emotional health (see Chapter 4, "T'ai Chi Expands the Mind and Lightens the Heart"). T'ai Chi has been called an inner-cise because it uniquely focuses the mind on the internal condition of the body rather than on an external performance. Therefore, whereas practicing baseball makes you better at baseball and playing ping pong makes you a better ping pong player, T'ai Chi practice makes you better at everything you do.

Advantages of Innercise

T'ai Chi improves our overall performance on a physical level because it provides us with a daily picture of how we operate. Through its slow deliberate movements we can, with a kind of inner sight, see inside ourselves to observe breath, posture, and tension levels. This allows us to correct problems before they become illnesses or injuries.

Some athletes have used medication to hide pain. T'ai Chi is the opposite of a painkiller. T'ai Chi helps us become aware of problems *before* they become acute. We do not want to hide pain because pain is the body's way of telling us that some part of us needs healing attention. However, as T'ai Chi and QiGong help the body get that gentle healing attention, they also help relieve chronic pain conditions. So T'ai Chi and QiGong help to heal injuries or illnesses that pain alerts us to, but they also help us deal with the pain as those conditions are allowed to heal. Painkillers, on the other hand, separate our mind from our body and neither heal nor grant us the awareness needed to avoid further injuries.

Ouch

On pain medication, T'ai Chi realizes there are no absolutes. When pain medication is needed, it is a wonderful thing to have and should be used. No one should force themselves to be in agony need-lessly. However, if QiGong and T'ai Chi can help reduce the need for pain medication, or help prevent injury that might result in that need, it is a very healthy option.

Having said that, if you have an existing condition causing acute pain, the pain may be so debilitating or distracting that other therapies like T'ai Chi and QiGong are impossible to attempt. This is not an either or situation. Use medication as needed and use T'ai Chi and QiGong as needed. The two can work in concert to help you recover. As always, discuss this with your doctor.

T'ai Chi tones the muscles, increases breathing capacity, lowers stress levels, improves organ function and corrects poor posture. All these things help the body maximize its self-healing potential, which will be discussed in Chapter 3, "Medical T'ai Chi: The Prescription for the Future."

Problems with Outercise

We in the West suffer from the delusion that we can get our bodies fit, or even get our lives in order, without our minds being involved. For example, if you go to the health club, they will most likely have televisions above the stationary bikes or the stair climbing machines. The idea is that we can get healthy, lose stress, and get "buns of steel" while having our minds bombarded with CNN visions of world problems or the top 10 songs blasting in our ears. Of course we can get buns-of-steel, but we can't get *truly* healthy that way. We've erroneously equated a hard body with health. From my personal experience, I've found that an over emphasis on the development of muscles, built up to look good to the outer world and not necessarily for health reasons, can interfere with my energy flow and natural health processes. The slow mindful exercises of T'ai Chi give me a healthy muscle tone and also seem to support my immune system function so I get sick less. This should come as a great relief to anyone who is tired of the nausea of hot, sweaty, bone pounding exercise routines.

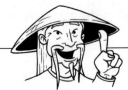

Sage Sifu Says

The Taoist philosopher, Lao Tzu, recognized that over-conditioning just to look good to the outside world would not produce the desired result of health.

Stretch a bow out all the way,
  And you'll regret that you didn't stop in time.
Sharpen a sword to its finest edge,
  And the edge will break very quickly.
Rest when you've achieved your goal,
  This is the way of heaven.

In other words, if you drive yourself to pump up your muscles, you'll likely not stick with an exercise program, because its goal is in excess of your health needs. It's easier and wiser to do an exercise to make you healthy, rather than just to *look good*. This is what T'ai Chi is all about.

T'ai Chi Cleanses Tissue and Lymph Glands

Overemphasizing our outer appearance is a yang obsession and can discount our internal, or yin, needs. T'ai Chi's goal is balance, and regular practice can help achieve this balance as T'ai Chi healthfully tones muscles, while attending to internal needs as well. T'ai Chi encourages us to find quiet and stillness of the mind so that our nervous system can begin to cleanse itself of accumulated thoughts and worries. This allows a deep tissue cleansing by encouraging deep relaxation and full breath, which lets the accumulated toxins in muscles release into the body's natural cleansing systems. Our body actually holds onto anxiety in a chemical form called "lactic acids," and T'ai Chi's deep releases help cleanse that and other toxins from the body. The gentle massage of T'ai Chi movement also begins to clear the lymph glands.

T'ai Chi gives you the best of both worlds. T'ai Chi can make you more gorgeous on the outside, even as it beautifies your "terrific personality."

T'ai Chi and Weight Loss

T'ai Chi can be a powerful addition to the many healthy and effective weight loss programs there are to choose from. Furthermore, T'ai Chi can help move the emphasis away from the external perception of judging negatively how you look or what you weigh, and put that emphasis on nurturing who you are (thin or heavy). By ignoring this, some fad diets only promote temporary reductions in calories rather than deep or lasting lifestyle changes. However, T'ai Chi can be a powerful ally to the many quality weight loss programs that do attend to self image issues, for the following reasons.

T'ai Chi works from the inside out. It promotes self-acceptance and self-nurturing. As you care more for yourself, you are drawn toward activities and foods that nurture your existence. T'ai Chi is a gradual healthy program of life change that encourages rather than demands or restricts, causing some deep internal part of yourself to draw you more effortlessly toward behavioral changes. T'ai Chi does not compete with healthy weight loss programs, but actually may significantly expedite their benefit and improve your chances of sticking with them.T'ai Chi burns about 280 calories per hour, surprisingly providing, despite its slow and gentle pace, many of the immediate results gained from other exercises. To put this in perspective, realize that downhill skiing burns only 350 calories per hour, making T'ai Chi nearly as effective in calorie consumption. Moreover, T'ai Chi is very safe, low impact, takes no equipment, and can be performed in the conference room at work during break time or even in the bathroom when you sneak off for an unofficial stress break.

The great feeling that comes from doing T'ai Chi is a terrific incentive to keep you coming back to it again and again. T'ai Chi gives you that "special time" alone for yourself to just enjoy how your body feels as it lets go of stress and relaxes. This makes

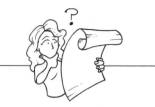

Know Your Chinese

Yin and **yang** are the Chinese concepts of universal forces. All things are an eternally flowing interaction of two opposites; the ideal is healthy balance in all things. Yin is internal; yang is external. Yin is dark; yang is light. Yin is feminine; yang is masculine. Yin is passive receptive; yang is dynamic and expressive. Even food has yin and yang qualities, so this balance determines a healthy diet.

it a much easier routine to stick with. And the good feelings it promotes in your body help you learn to love your body more and to accept it the way it is. Surprisingly, the more we accept the way we are now, the easier it is to change to the way we want to be.

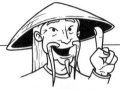

Sage Sifu Says

Even though T'ai Chi promotes healthy weight loss, remember not to hold on tightly to a desired outcome. T'ai Chi is always most effective when we do it for the simple enjoyment of how it feels. Let everything else be an unexpected surprise.

Another powerful component to T'ai Chi's affect on weight loss is how it helps us let go of stress and nervous tension. Much of our evening snacking is "nervous snacking." This is an attempt to repress feelings of unease by stimulating our taste buds and other sensations. That's why we usually want really greasy, salty, or sweet foods to munch on at night when we are trying not to feel our stress; the strong tastes distract our minds.

Yet, T'ai Chi does even more to promote healthy weight loss. T'ai Chi's physical, emotional, and mental centering helps us feel very pleasant. The Chinese call this state "smooth Qi," while modern psychologists call it "homeostasis." But no matter what you call it, it feels good. As T'ai Chi and QiGong get us more and more in the habit of "feeling good," we become more aware of what habits reinforce that lovely feeling. We then begin to realize that certain junk foods take us away from our feelings of smooth Qi. We also begin to understand in deep ways that proper sleep, diet, and making time to enjoy life all contribute to our smooth Qi. The more we feel that way, the more we want to feel that way. This helps our body to find a healthy weight effortlessly as we learn to love things that promote this feeling, such as light healthy foods and our T'ai Chi and QiGong.

T'ai Chi Tones Muscles, Too

Not only does T'ai Chi tone muscles but it does so while promoting a more elegant elongated form. Many exercises are designed to "buff us up," giving us a shorter, stockier appearance. T'ai Chi, on the other hand, may actually lengthen the body over time, making us more lithe. As we age, it is our tension that shortens our bodies more than gravity. By practicing T'ai Chi's relaxed movements every day, we allow the muscles to release tension as they seemingly let go of one another and release their grip on the bones and connective tissue. We can actually lengthen each time we do T'ai Chi.

T'ai Chi Oils the Joints

As we age we often lose mobility, feeling like the rusty Tin Man in the Wizard of Oz. In fact, this "rusting" can start at about any age; we need only to stop using our bodies fully. There are two reasons we lose mobility. The first is because calcium deposits that normal usage would wear off build up in our joints. The second is because our liquid systems function less well when we are sedentary. Therefore, our joints get more brittle and stiff.

Ouch!

Never force joints to be more mobile than feels good. T'ai Chi is more about being quiet enough to "hear" what the body tells you than about moving in any certain way. When doing T'ai Chi or anything else, be aware of your current limits. Then play at easing up against that limit day after day after day. You are limitless. Enjoy the ride!

T'ai Chi can solve both problems better than any other exercise. T'ai Chi movements require the body to rotate about 95 percent of the ways it can be rotated, thereby working out the potential calcium deposits wherever they may be lurking. No other Western exercise comes close to this. Swimming, for example, only rotates about 65 percent of the body's potential movement. Secondly, T'ai Chi stimulates the liquid systems of the body to keep our joints and other tissue more supple, even into advanced old age.

Steppin' Cool and Healthful

T'ai Chi's attention to posture really improves your grace, whether you want to move like Grace Kelly or Gene Kelly. Plus, as T'ai Chi smoothes your moves, it also heals your body.

T'ai Chi recognizes that the body always wants to be in the best, most healthful posture. However, our tension sometimes wrenches the bones or vertebrae out of place. This causes pain and eventually physical damage, not only to the back, but also to associated organs because all parts of the body are affected by spinal alignment.

By practicing T'ai Chi and QiGong each day, the muscles seem to begin releasing their tight grip on the bones, which can relieve pressure on the vertebrae caused by muscle tension. This allows the spine to realign, along with other bones and joints. You will be more graceful, more spry and energetic, and more charming because you will have less and less chronic pain.

T'ai Chi's Like a Day at the Spa, Without the Bill

Like a day at the spa, T'ai Chi leaves you with a healthful glow caused by increased circulation, energy flow, and the resulting nourishment of each cell of the body, including skin. The beauty salons of the future will provide access to these exercises (some already do). T'ai Chi can help you feel as though you spent everyday at the spa, except your credit card won't feel the pain.

Yet, ultimately T'ai Chi allows us to achieve the only real beauty. The beauty of being a real and caring human being.

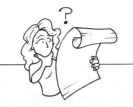

Know Your Chinese

Dan tien is an energy center located slightly below the navel inside the body. In T'ai Chi, it is known to be the center of gravity, and all T'ai Chi movement is directed by this point, while the torso and limbs are extensions of this central point.

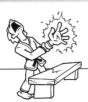

Ouch!

The old adage "lift with your legs, not your back" is a modern version of T'ai Chi's admonition to "move from the dan tien." T'ai Chi makes you very safety conscious. Yet, this awareness of how to move, push, and lift in ways that don't hurt you will become almost instinct as you practice T'ai Chi over the years.

Dan Tien Is the Physical Center of T'ai Chi and You

T'ai Chi provides us with much more overall energy during the day and much more power for specific tasks. It does this by getting us to quiet our minds enough to become aware of the way we move and of our postural alignment while we are moving.

T'ai Chi movements are done by focusing our awareness on two things. Our dan tien, or center of gravity, is located about 1½ to 3 inches below the navel near the center of the body—our vertical axis, or our line of posture. In the hard martial arts like karate, they know of the power of the dan tien. The ability to exert extreme force for breaking boards and bricks comes from awareness of moving from the center of our body, which is the dan tien. But again, that same power can help us lift our laundry basket or turn over our mattress with much less chance of hurting our back or pulling a muscle. For those who have some physical problem, awareness of dan tien may make you more capable of simply functioning more normally again.

Dan Tien Is Expressive Power

No matter what form our physical expression takes, the internal self-awareness of moving from and breathing into the dan tien will add power. Whether you are making a board room presentation, ironing the clothes, or running a marathon, your performance will be simultaneously more effortless and much more powerful.

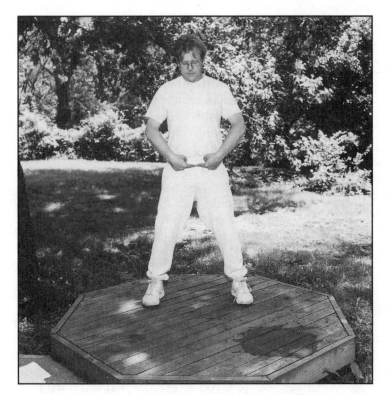

The dan tien is located about 1¹/₂ to 3 inches below the navel, near the center of the body, although slightly toward the front.

All great coaches know that real power comes from the dan tien. Even if they have never heard of the term, they all know that dan tien is the source of expressive power. Singing or acting coaches talk of "speaking from the diaphragm," golf coaches speak of "swinging with the belly button," and baseball coaches teach batters to "squash the bug," which is another way of saying to swing with the pelvis by pivoting the back foot as if squishing a bug. But, no matter how they describe it, they all are saying that any great athletic performance or physical expression is powered by centering the movement from the dan tien.

Moving from Dan Tien Is Effortless

Becoming aware of the dan tien means moving from the core of your physical being. Remember playing with spinning tops as a child? If you put your hands on the outside edge of the top and tried to spin it, it was a lot of work, and it didn't spin very much. However, once you learned to place your thumb and forefinger around the center spindle of the top, you found that just a little flick of the thumb and finger sent the top spinning like mad. This is what moving from the dan tien is all about. This is why moving from dan tien makes a boxer's punch harder, a golfer's swing more powerful, and a lawn mower's job easier, and easier on the back.

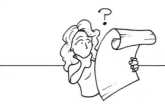

Know Your Chinese

Soong Yi-Dien! (pronounced *shoong yee-dee-en*) is often heard in Hong Kong's famous garment district. It means "the suit is too tight, loosen it up, loosen it up!" Our bodies are our mind's suits, and we are all wearing our suits way too tight. Chinese T'ai Chi masters will therefore say, "Soong Yi-Dien" as well.

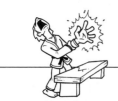

Ouch

Whenever you catch yourself trying too hard or notice your head and shoulder muscles tightening...just stop. Take a few breaths and on each sighing exhale, let the world roll off your shoulders. It is amazing how well the world holds itself up each time your bony little shoulders take a break. Take more breaks from holding the world up.

As T'ai Chi teaches us to move from the dan tien, it also helps us realize that we can let most of our muscles relax while the dan tien moves us around our harried lives. At first this concept of effortless movement sounds odd, but with practice, as you get better and better at it, it makes sense. The more we allow the body to relax, the more the raw power of the dan tien's movement comes through in our golfing, housework, or verbal and physical communication.

When our bodies are tight, the power of the dan tien is watered down. Even if a baseball batter squashes the bug well and swings with his pelvis or dan tien, if his arms and shoulders are tight, the dan tien's power can't flow through them. So, to maximize the power of dan tien, we must also teach the body to relax enough to allow that power to pour up through the arms or down through the legs.

Knowing that relaxing our body increases our power does not automatically translate into increased power. In fact, trying to memorize too many of T'ai Chi's benefits will tighten you up. Let this information wash over you effortlessly. Chapter 11, "Sitting QiGong (Jing Gong)," will give you an exercise that will teach your body how to be effortless. In Part 3, you will learn how QiGong will relax your mind, which will in turn relax your body. This maximizes the expression of whatever magic we are here in this world to express by allowing dan tien's power to flow through us unimpeded by tension. T'ai Chi's practice of moving from the dan tien makes T'ai Chi a great athletic trainer. Therefore, QiGong's ability to help us release the tension inhibiting dan tien's power makes QiGong perhaps the world's greatest self-improvement program. Come back and reread this chapter after practicing the Sitting QiGong exercise in Part 3. This will help you see how T'ai Chi incorporates powerful health and performance tools into not only your way of moving, but also your way of thinking and living.

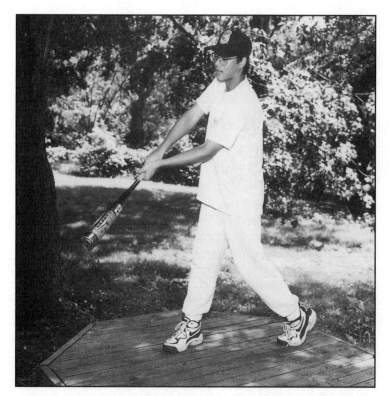

This photo illustrates how a loose frame sends the full force of the dan tien's motion up through the body, out the bat, and into the ball. Note that the batter's back foot "squashing the bug" sends the dan tien into motion toward the ball.

Stay Loose, Bruiser!

The goal of T'ai Chi is to move through life as effortlessly as possible. This doesn't mean we run from challenge and adventure. T'ai Chi teaches us to breathe easily and relax, no matter how much adventure we are going through. However, as we practice T'ai Chi, we may find that some of the negative drama in our lives is self-created; as we let go of unnecessary stress, we will likely find more calm. This will save our energy for adventures that are really fun.

So, T'ai Chi teaches us to let the body let go of itself. We use only the muscles that are absolutely necessary for each movement, thereby conserving energy for when we really need it.

The most beautiful way to express this concept is found in a French fencing (sword fighting) term. The French fencing masters speak of how you should hold the foil, or sword. *"Hold it lightly like a dove, so not to crush it in your grip, and yet firmly so it does not fly away."* This is the lesson for life that T'ai Chi brings to mind and body again and again, and powerfully affects how we view our world. If we hold onto possessions or loved ones too tightly, it will reflect in our muscles, health, and our relationships. We will squeeze all the magic out of life, just like we can squeeze all the power out of our sports performance. This is why great sports heroes never hold onto the idea of a championship; they just relax into the moment.

The Dan Tien Improves All Activity

In T'ai Chi we move and think from the dan tien, the center of physical gravity. This also centers our awareness and maximizes the power of any physical effort. As T'ai Chi teaches us to loosen, breathe, and enjoy, everything we do improves.

T'ai Chi's and QiGong's mental centering of our awareness in the dan tien area is coupled with a feeling of flowing energy (see Part 3). This cleanses our nervous system of all cloudiness and distortion, clearing communication between mind and body. By focusing our awareness within and letting go of the stress of the day, we become more focused on what we are doing right here and right now. So, if we are hitting a golf ball right here and right now, or cooking dinner, or making a speech at the PTA meeting, we will be more likely to make a record drive, a spectacular meal, or an inspired speech.

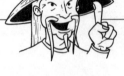

Sage Sifu Says

The facts and figures on the benefits of T'ai Chi are valuable only if they encourage you to stick with it. The benefits of T'ai Chi and QiGong come pleasantly and effortlessly by breathing, relaxing, and celebrating the miracle of your physical body.

T'ai Chi vs. Yoga

Students always ask what the difference between yoga and T'ai Chi is. When Jay Leno's character on The Tonight Show, "Iron Jay," was asked that question he said, "T'ai Chi, dat's a little spicier den yoga, *ain't it?*"

Without tackling which is spicier, let's begin by looking at what makes them similar. Both T'ai Chi and yoga are excellent mind/body fitness tools that are being practiced by more and more people around the world. Both help us let go of stress and cultivate a sense of well being in our lives. Both can be very gentle and used by almost anyone.

Now, some differences. T'ai Chi is more easily practiced by those in wheel chairs because T'ai Chi is done upright, whereas many yoga positions require lying down. T'ai Chi's standing motion continually challenges our balance, which explains why T'ai Chi is the best balance conditioner in the world. And, since it is done standing up, T'ai Chi can be performed about anywhere outdoors. Furthermore, T'ai Chi can be practiced in any type of clothing, making it much more convenient for corporate settings. While yoga postures are often static poses, T'ai Chi's postures flow one into the other, just as life's changes flow one into the other, making T'ai Chi's effortless changes a model for life.

While yoga is practiced to prepare the body to experience a blissful meditative state, with T'ai Chi, the QiGong meditative state is often practiced *before* movements. This is because T'ai Chi's goal is to bring the blissful state of enlightened awareness into our physical lives. Yoga goes to a place of peace, T'ai Chi brings that place of peace into our daily activities. Both are wonderful habits and can each enhance the effectiveness of the other. I recommend yoga highly.

T'ai Chi and yoga are complementary disciplines, and your T'ai Chi practice may prepare you to dip your toe into yoga, or vice versa. There are strengths that both offer uniquely, and although I advocate making T'ai Chi a part of your daily life, I encourage you to try yoga as well. Life is a great experiment.

The Least You Need to Know

➤ T'ai Chi tones, beautifies, and empowers you and everything you do.

➤ T'ai Chi done wisely does no damage to your body and can help keep it working for as long as you need it.

➤ By teaching self acceptance, T'ai Chi makes you more adventurous in life.

➤ T'ai Chi can enhance athletic training, no matter what your game.

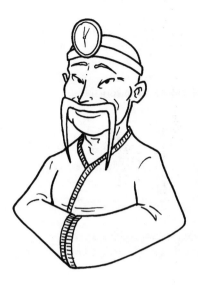

Chapter 3

Medical T'ai Chi: The Prescription for the Future

The doctor of the future will prescribe no medicine, but will interest his patients in the care of the human frame...

—Thomas Alva Edison

T'ai Chi and QiGong's medical benefits have been studied for nearly 2,000 years in China and for only about 20 years in the West. However, Western medical research is rapidly discovering what Chinese medicine has long realized, that T'ai Chi provides more medical benefits than any other single exercise. That's why this ancient Chinese exercise is at the cutting edge of modern medical research.

This chapter will give you both an understanding of how Chinese medicine views our health and also the emerging Western scientific research that validates these ancient views. The bottom line is we are very lucky to live at a time when these wonderful tools are available to us in the West. We are also lucky to be able to see scientific proof that they work because as practitioners of Traditional Chinese Medicine understood centuries ago, our faith is the greatest healer. So, if we know in our minds that T'ai Chi works, our bodies will allow it to do its magic, and we will be the big winner.

We live in a stressful world; only recently has Western medical research come to recognize that stress is at the root of most health problems. Therefore, the health crisis that stress is causing in the West has actually created a great opportunity for us because it is opening us up to the wonders of Traditional Chinese Medicine and tools like T'ai Chi and QiGong. In fact, the list of T'ai Chi's measurable health benefits below indicates how this opening to T'ai Chi may save us from our health care crisis. T'ai Chi can:

➤ Boost the immune system

➤ Slow the aging process

➤ Reduce anxiety, depression, and overall mood disturbance

➤ Lower high blood pressure

➤ Alleviate stress responses

➤ Enhance the body's natural healing powers such as recovering from injury

➤ Increase breathing capacity

➤ Reduce asthma and allergy reactions

The Chinese character for "crisis" is a combination of two other characters. One for "danger" and the other for "opportunity."

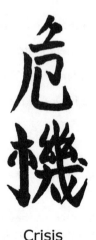

Crisis

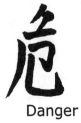

Danger

Danger + Opportunity = Crisis

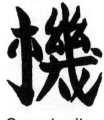

Opportunity

➤ Improve balance and coordination TWICE as well as the best balance conditioning exercises in the world

➤ Help to ensure full range mobility far into old age

➤ Provide the lowest impact weight-bearing exercise known

Mind Over Matter

T'ai Chi's artful beauty can make us forget that it is actually one of the most highly evolved health technologies on Earth. The Chinese realized that our mind or consciousness is the root of who we are. Our health and our lives are merely reflections of our state of mind. Therefore, T'ai Chi's mindful quality incorporates the mind and body into a powerful healing force.

Interestingly, Western science now sees that Traditional Chinese Medicine's ancient insights were right on the money. A new science called *psychoneuroimmunology* has found that our mind constantly communicates to every cell of our body.

Emotional chemicals, known as neuropeptides, flow throughout our bodies, communicating every feeling to the entire body. So, when hitting every red light on the street aggravates us or we become anxious in every line we stand in, we walk around in a state of perpetual panic (or as Bruce Springsteen sang, "Yer life is one long emergency"). This negatively affects our heart, brain, and entire circulatory system. In fact, those effects in turn affect other organs, which can cause a breakdown of the entire system over time, causing, for example, kidney failure, heart enlargement, and hardening of the arteries.

But, don't fret, T'ai Chi helps us do just the opposite. We can decide to let issues slide right off us, literally breathing fears out with every sigh and yawn. As we sit in QiGong meditation or move in T'ai Chi's soothing postures, we let a nourishing healing flow of Qi, or life energy, fill every cell of our bodies.

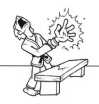

Ouch

Before adding T'ai Chi to your physical therapy program, consult your physician to see if T'ai Chi might affect your medication levels. For example, many with high blood pressure find their blood pressure lowers. Your physician should know if T'ai Chi can alter your current therapy for such conditions and then can lower your medication safely.

T'ai Sci

Psychoneuroimmunology is a modern science studying how the mind's attitudes and beliefs affect our physical health. *Psycho* means mind, *neuro* means nervous system, and *immunology* means system of health defenses.

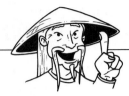

Sage Sifu Says

Traditional Chinese Medicine (TCM) differs from the Western approach in that its focus is holistic. *Holistic* means it views the body as an integrated whole. A TCM doctor does not treat only symptoms, but rather tries to discover the root of health problems.

For example, if we have allergy problems, Western pharmaceuticals might send chemical missiles in to dry out the sinuses. This does stop the runny nose, but some medications may result in irritating the surrounding tissue by drying it out, or in other undesirable side effects. Acupuncture on the other hand, or T'ai Chi in the long run, will enable the body's natural balancing to occur, reducing the incidence of sinus problems in a way that nurtures the tissue. This is done by reestablishing the blocked flow of Qi that is at the root of the problem.

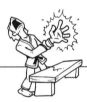

Ouch

Don't try too hard to memorize any of these details on Traditional Chinese or Western medicine. Rather, let the concepts wash over your relaxed mind. The important stuff will stick, and you can always go back to look up details later.

To fully appreciate T'ai Chi's medical benefits, it may be helpful to understand how Traditional Chinese Medicine views the body.

Traditional Chinese Medicine has known for centuries what Western science is only now discovering: that our mind and body are two inseparable things. In Traditional Chinese Medicine, there is a joke that "the only place the mind, body, emotions, and spirit are separate is in textbooks." In real life and T'ai Chi, it just isn't so. T'ai Chi's slow mindful movements are the epitome of this union of mind and body.

So, when your body's muscles are rigid, your thinking will likely be more rigid, too. Likewise, if your thinking is harsh and rigid, this will in time be reflected in stiffness in your muscular frame. This stiffness impedes the flow of Qi, which diminishes our health. Therefore, your mind and your thoughts have as much, or maybe more, to do with your health than the food you eat or the exercise you get.

Energy meridians link all the organs and the entire physical body to the mind and emotional systems. This explains how T'ai Chi and QiGong's mind/body exercises integrate all aspects of the self into a powerful self-healing system.

What Are Energy Meridians?

What are these energy meridians that T'ai Chi helps to unblock? By now you know that Qi flows through and powers every cell in your body, the way electricity powers your house. Without Qi, the cell would be dead, for Qi is the life force. The meridians are how Qi gets to the cells. You can't see these meridians; you can only detect the energy that moves through them, just as you cannot see an ocean current in the water, but you can detect its motion.

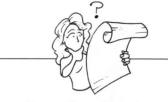

Know Your Chinese

The energy meridians are known as **jing luo**. Jing literally means "to move through," and luo means "a net." So energy meridians are a network of channels.

There are ancient maps of these meridians, made thousands of years ago by Traditional Chinese doctors. These acupuncture meridian maps show 14 main energy meridians that carry Qi throughout the body internally and externally. The names follow, listed first by the modern acupuncture abbreviation, then by the English name, and a few followed by the Chinese name in italics.

- ➤ CV = Conception Vessel or *Ren Mai*
- ➤ CX = Pericardium Channel
- ➤ GB = Gallbladder Channel
- ➤ GV = Governing Vessel or *Du Mai*
- ➤ HE = Heart Channel
- ➤ KI = Kidney Channel
- ➤ LI = Large Intestine
- ➤ LU = Lung Channel
- ➤ LV = Liver Channel
- ➤ SI = Small Intestine Channel
- ➤ SP = Spleen-Pancreas Channel
- ➤ ST = Stomach Channel
- ➤ TW = Triple Warmer or *San Jiao* Channel
- ➤ UB = Urinary Bladder Channel

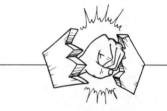

A T'ai Chi Punch Line

There are also acupuncture maps for animals. In fact, some racing horses have their own personal acupuncturists. Many veterinarians are beginning to use acupuncture as part of their practice.

Acupuncture and T'ai Chi

There are three aspects of Traditional Chinese Medicine: acupuncture, herbal medicine, and T'ai Chi/QiGong. All three share a common premise that Qi pours through the body, and our health is diminished when the energy flow gets blocked.

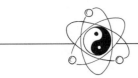

T'ai Sci

Modern acupuncturists often call the Qi meridians bioenergetic circuits.

So, whether an acupuncturist is treating you with needles, an herbalist is prescribing herbs, or you are practicing T'ai Chi, you are trying to balance the imbalances, or unblock the energy that flows throughout your body. Millions of Americans are now using alternative therapies like acupuncture and herbs. If you practice T'ai Chi daily, your relaxed state will help herbs or acupuncture work even more effectively.

The energy meridians, which flow throughout the interior of the body, have 361 points that surface at the skin, and these are the most common treatment points acupuncturists use. But the whole body and even the mind can be treated with acupuncture because these meridians that surface at the skin also flow inside the body, through the brain and organs.

T'ai Chi and QiGong affect the same energy flow that acupuncture does, although acupuncture can be better for acute problems, whereas T'ai Chi is a daily tune-up. Therefore, acupuncturists often recommend T'ai Chi to their patients, and T'ai Chi teachers recommend acupuncture to students with chronic or acute conditions, as a supplement to the students' standard medical treatments. T'ai Chi and acupuncture are very complimentary, and each makes the other more effective.

An example of an acupuncture meridian map. This also comes in a three-dimensional model.

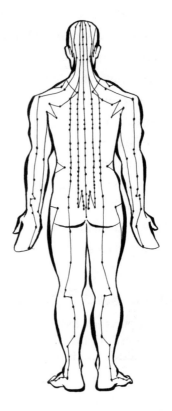

Say, "OOOOHHHHHMMMMMM"—OHM Meter That Is

It is mind boggling when you consider that many modern acupuncturists find acupuncture points with electronic equipment, not unlike an Ohmmeter. What's amazing is that acupuncture maps were made long before electronics was developed, some believe over 2,000 years ago.

How did they know where those points were back then? They may have felt them. As you practice T'ai Chi and QiGong, you will eventually begin to feel the Qi flowing from your hands or in your body.

T'ai Chi Is Footloose and Healthfully

Acupuncture sees the body holistically, meaning that each small part of the body contains connections to the whole body. Therefore, an acupuncturist can treat any problem in the whole body through, for example, the ears. Likewise, any part of the body, or even the mind, can be treated through the hands or the feet.

One of the powerful health benefits T'ai Chi provides is a daily acupuncture tune-up. Because T'ai Chi is so slow and the weight shifts so deliberate, with the body very relaxed, the feet are massaged by the earth during a T'ai Chi exercise. The bottoms of the feet have acupuncture points that affect the entire body, and yes the mind, too. Acupressure is acupuncture without the needles. So the foot massage is a 20-minute T'ai Chi session that stimulates all the acupuncture points on the foot through acupressure, thereby treating the whole body. No other exercise provides this type of slow, relaxed motion, making T'ai Chi unique in providing you an acupuncture tune-up each time you do your daily exercise.

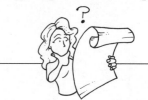

Know Your Chinese

Zang-Fu literally translated means "solid-hollow." Organs within the body considered to be hollow, like the stomach or large intestines, are Fu organs. While the solid organs, such as liver and lung, are Zang organs.

Don't Be Zang Fu-lish

Another profound benefit T'ai Chi provides is a gentle massaging of the internal organs. Because T'ai Chi moves the body in about 95 percent of the possible motions it can go through, it not only clears the joints of calcium deposits, but it also gently massages the internal organs.

In Traditional Chinese Medicine (TCM), this is a powerful therapy for optimum health. TCM recognizes that the body is an integrated whole whereby all the parts are connected by the flow of Qi. In fact, the Chinese system of medicine is built upon a Zang Fu graph, which shows how organs interact with and depend on one another for good healthy function.

The energy flow affects different organs through the Sheng Cycle and the Ko cycle. This shows how organs are interactive and interdependent on one another for healthful function.

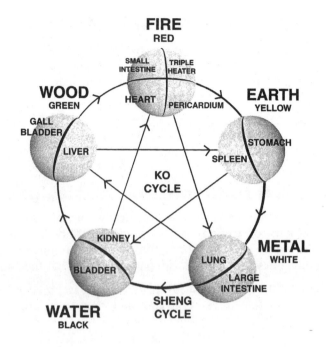

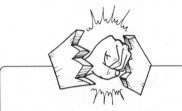

A T'ai Chi Punch Line

The Zang Fu system uses a memory model, applying each organ to one of the five elements of the Earth. The Chinese see the world as made of Earth, Metal, Water, Wood, and Fire. See the Zang Fu chart for which organs go with which element.

Therefore, because T'ai Chi massages all the organs through its gentle full rotations, it helps to balance all the integrating activities of the Zang Fu systems.

T'ai Chi and QiGong Benefit Emotions

Acupuncture, herbal medicine, and T'ai Chi/QiGong use the Zang Fu system to understand how the body, mind, and emotions integrate. A problem with a particular organ may have emotional symptoms. Likewise, a chronic emotional state may have a physical impact on the organs. The following chart illustrates the Zang Fu connection between organs and emotions commonly related to imbalances with those organs or their energy channels.

➤ Liver = Depression, anger

➤ Heart = Excess joy (such as manic behavior), excess mental function

➤ Spleen = Obsession

➤ Lung = Anguish, grief, melancholy

➤ Kidney = Fear, fright

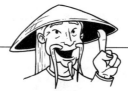

Sage Sifu Says

If you go to a Traditional Chinese Physician, he or she may likely ask you about your emotions as well as your physical symptoms because emotional states may help lead them to understand which organ's energy is deficient or in excess.

So, T'ai Chi benefits the mental and emotional states, not only by encouraging us to let go of the day's problems by focusing on breath and movement, but in other ways as well. T'ai Chi stimulates the organs with gentle massage, while stimulating the acupressure points on the feet and throughout the body, with its gentle relaxed postures. The breathing in T'ai Chi is full, yet effortless, encouraging internal releases of mental and emotional blocks that also help the internal Zang Fu systems become less restricted, more free flowing, and healthful on mental, emotional, and physical levels. Chapter 4 will explain how T'ai Chi and QiGong can provide mental and emotional healing.

T'ai Chi and QiGong Increase Flexibility

T'ai Chi not only increases flexibility by regularly stretching the muscles very gently, but through the Zang Fu system as well. As we age, especially but not exclusively men, we often find a depletion in our kidney energy. The kidney energy is responsible for the function of the liquid systems of the body. Therefore, the decrease in kidney energy that accompanies aging causes our connective tissue, such as tendons, to become brittle.
We are then much more likely to tear, or otherwise injure, our bones or joints when we stumble or fall.

So, the tremendous balance improvements T'ai Chi offers are only part of why T'ai Chi practitioners are much less likely than other people to suffer falling injuries. The improved performance of all organ functions enhances the entire physical body's health. In fact, in this way, sitting QiGong may also increase flexibility, even though it is a nonphysical exercise.

Western Medicine's Research on T'ai Chi and QiGong

After reading this section you should be satisfied beyond a doubt that *T'ai Chi works*. So when you get to the QiGong and T'ai Chi exercises later in Parts 3, 4, and 5, you won't have to think about their benefits. The mind is the greatest healer. Therefore, if you believe in the value of your therapy, it will be much more effective for you.

Stress Is the Symptom

By now you know that stress is the chief cause of illness in the modern world. As Western medicine discovers that T'ai Chi and QiGong are effective stress-reducing exercises, these powerful mind/body health tools are being used in more and more hospitals and are prescribed by more and more doctors.

Studies show that reaction to stress can damage the entire body. It causes chronic hypertension (high blood pressure), which can cause the arteries to harden, kidney damage, and enlargement of the heart. Stress also has been shown to impair our ability to think and actually shrinks the hypothalamus and the hypocampus parts of the brain. Yikes!!

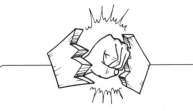

A T'ai Chi Punch Line

Traditional Chinese Medicine sees the body and mind intertwined. So, a rigid body can cause us to think rigidly as well. Or perhaps more accurately a rigid mind can cause us to have a rigid body.

Who Ya Gonna Call?

T'ai Chi is the stress buster. An article in *Occupational Therapy Week* explains that T'ai Chi's emphasis on posture and diaphragmatic breathing (breathing from your diaphragm) accounts for a practitioner's reduction in muscular tension and the stress it causes. Patients using T'ai Chi report a greater ability to cope with fear and anxiety, as that physical relaxation is reflected in their mental attitude.

Bellevue Psychiatric Hospital in New York City provided T'ai Chi to both staff and patients. Their Activity Therapy Supervisor said, "T'ai Chi is a natural and safe vehicle to *neutralize* rather than resist the stress in our personal lives, an ability which we greatly need to nurture in our modern fast-paced society."

T'ai Chi Is Your Heart's Best Friend

Harvard Medical School's *Women's Health Watch Journal* reported that, "T'ai Chi has *salubrious* effects," and that "practicing T'ai Chi regularly may delay the decline of cardiopulmonary function in older adults…T'ai Chi was found to be as effective as meditation in reducing stress hormones."

A Duke University study recently announced that managing stress controls heart disease even more effectively than exercise. Since T'ai Chi provides both powerful stress management and gentle exercise, T'ai Chi is your heart's very best friend. Now, go out and play nice with your new friend.

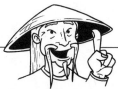

Sage Sifu Says

With all these T'ai Chi and QiGong facts swimming through your mind, now is a good time to practice QiGong's mind clearing tools. Take a deep breath from your abdomen to your chest, and on the sighing exhale, let your shoulders relax away from your neck as they sink towards the floor. Repeat this several times, and as you release the breath, imagine that every cell in your body is relaxing as you release each breath. Now as you let go of the breath, let all your cranial muscles release their grip on your skull, and as you let go, allow your mind to release all the facts and figures it is trying to remember.

Ironically, you will find that the more your mind lets go of trying to hold onto facts, the more easily it can absorb information.

T'ai Chi Reduces Mental Stress

A study cited in the *Journal of Psychosomatic Research* claimed T'ai Chi study subjects reported less tension, depression, anger, fatigue, confusion, and anxiety; they felt more vigorous and, in general, had less total mood disturbance.

The *Journal of Black Psychology* states that many African-Americans suffer from chronic high blood pressure. The article explains that hypertension is a physical result of psychological stress. The article proposes T'ai Chi as a holistic way for treating psychosomatic illnesses, or those illnesses caused by stress.

T'ai Chi may also help us think better. Research has shown that stress can limit the development of the hypocampus, the part of the brain that deals with learning and memory. So, T'ai Chi's ability to reduce stress responses may actually enhance our ability to learn and remember.

T'ai Chi Lowers Body Stress

Working Woman magazine's article on T'ai Chi said, "increasingly mind/body workouts are replacing high-impact aerobics, and other body punishing exercises of the 1980s.

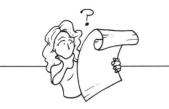

Know Your Chinese

T'ai Chi and QiGong have long been known to boost the immune system. Ancient Chinese medicine understood the concept of the immune system, which the Chinese called **bu qi**, **bu xue**, meaning tonify the Qi and blood. When Qi and blood are strengthened, we are better able to fight off infection and disease.

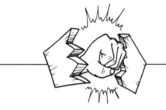

A T'ai Chi Punch Line

I was once studying T'ai Chi and QiGong in Hong Kong. Because of the time difference, I was waking up at 3 am. With nothing else to do, I became a particularly diligent student and practiced Gathering Qi or Standing Post for nearly an hour and a half each morning. After about a week of this, I began to visually see the Qi flowing around people. Especially their heads.

I noticed that those who seemed to be enjoying the day had large pluming expanses of energy around them, while those appearing driven and stressed had tiny restricted energy emanating from them.

These mind/body workouts are kinder to the joints and muscles and can reduce the tension that often contributes to the development of disease, which makes them especially appropriate for high-powered, stressed-out baby boomers."

T'ai Chi Boosts Your Immune System

Prevention magazine reported a study on T'ai Chi's effects on the immune system. They found that regular practice of T'ai Chi may increase the body's production of T-Cells. These T-Cells are T-lymphocytes. "Lymphowhats???" you might ask. It doesn't matter. What matters is that these little T-Cells help the immune system destroy bacteria and possibly even tumor cells. If T'ai Chi can make more of these little buggers, what are we waiting for. Let's T'ai Chi one on!

Cancer, QiGong, and Our Immune System

In China, QiGong is commonly prescribed as an adjunct to chemotherapy and radiation. Studies indicate that when QiGong is combined with standard cancer treatments, favorable results are obtained, treating virtually all forms and stages of cancer. Part of the reason for this success is that QiGong helps patients feel less helpless. Studies show that feelings of self-empowerment can have powerful healing benefits on the course of almost any disease, including cancer.

How Does T'ai Chi Fight for the Immune System?

American QiGong master Ken Cohen has dubbed a hormone called DHEA the Health Hormone. In his book, *Qigong: The Art and Science of Chinese Energy Healing*, Mr. Cohen explains that this hormone is believed to be linked to Qi.

DHEA is short for dehydroepiandrosterone. Yeah, I know, *forget-about-it.* But don't forget that DHEA is related to youthfulness, less disease, and a more functional immune system.

According to Mr. Cohen, low DHEA levels have been directly linked to cancer, diabetes, obesity, hypertension, allergies, heart disease, and most autoimmune diseases.

When we are under a lot of stress, our body exhausts itself of this important hormone. Therefore, by practicing T'ai Chi, we can increase DHEA levels, thereby increasing our immune systems ability to fight whatever steps in the ring with it. Let's RUMBLE!!

T'ai Chi does two wonderful things to help us age healthfully:

➤ It maximizes the body's full potential to regenerate healthy cells, which actually slows the aging process.

➤ It promotes a deep self-acceptance and self-awareness, so that as our body goes through the challenges of aging, we are much better able to handle and adjust to those changes, both physically and emotionally.

DHEA and T'ai Chi, Back Together Again

DHEA, short for dehydroepiandrosterone, is also involved in the aging process. This hormone's levels tend to decline with age, but the decline is much worse when under chronic stress. Add natural aging and chronic stress, and you have an express train to an old body. However, our old friend T'ai Chi once again comes to the rescue. T'ai Chi's gentle movements and breathing techniques promote the serenity that can keep DHEA from being depleted.

Of course, the increased circulation of blood and Qi also fully oxygenate the skin, which provides nourishment to our outer beauty. The Zang Fu system's being balanced by T'ai Chi's stimulation of acupressure points and massage of the internal organs also moves the liquids and oils of the body to the tissue that needs them, further adding to our external beauty and internal health.

T'ai Sci

Free radicals are atoms with an extra electron that bounce around wreaking havoc throughout the body. We see this with our eyes as aging. The calming effects of T'ai Chi and QiGong not only affect the mind, but can also reduce the damage done by free radicals, thereby slowing the aging process.

Aging's Radical, Dude! (Free Radicals, That Is)

There is a pesky little *free radical* atom in your body called "super oxide" that causes the body to age. Not only does it cause wrinkles and age spots, but can also weaken cartilage and joints. In fact,

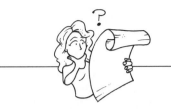

Know Your Chinese

Fan lao huan tong means "reverse old age and return to youthfulness." This is what the Chinese believe T'ai Chi and QiGong offer, and of course Western scientific methods are beginning to tell us how and why that happens. East meets West.

this super oxide may even induce cancer or other immune system disorders. *Obnoxious little things aren't they?*

However, regular T'ai Chi and QiGong practice can protect your body from these pesky free radicals by activating an enzyme called *superoxide dismutase* (or SOD). SOD is our cellular superman and defends our cells from the ornery super oxides that break down our health systems.

A study of those who practiced QiGong for a half-hour a day for one year showed that their levels of SOD increased dramatically compared to people not doing QiGong. Another study showed a large increase in SOD after only two months of QiGong practice.

Make No Bones About It, T'ai Chi Does Your Body Good

The National Institute of Mental Health released a study showing that women under chronic stress with depression had weaker bones than those in normal emotional states. In fact, the stressed/depressed women had the bones of 70-year-old women, even though they were only 40 years old.

T'ai Chi lessens the incidence of depression and the body's stress responses, and is a gentle weight bearing exercise. These abilities may make T'ai Chi the best thing you can do to keep your bones healthy, even into old age.

T'ai Sci

In a university study on balance, researchers were testing a rather expensive computer model designed to improve people's balance. The researchers were stunned to find that a simple inexpensive exercise called T'ai Chi was in some ways nearly twice as effective as the expensive computer model.

T'ai Chi Does an Incredible Balancing Act!

For aging Americans, the simple act of stumbling and falling can often be fatal. The sixth largest cause of death for older Americans is complications from falling injuries. This costs our country about $10 billion a year and causes tremendous suffering for older people. We are all paying for our nation's poor balance in human suffering and in higher healthcare and health insurance costs.

T'ai Chi was part of a balance study by Harvard, Yale, the Center for Disease Control, Washington University School of Medicine, and Emory University. T'ai Chi practitioners fell and injured themselves only half as much as those practicing other balance training. This is an amazing finding that can change the lives of older Americans.

Although many of us are not in the age group that is likely to suffer serious injury from falling, we can all benefit greatly by having better balance. Better balance puts much less stress on the body throughout the workday, and you will find that you have much more energy as T'ai Chi practice improves your balance.

T'ai Chi Is Dirt Cheap and Can Be Done on Grass, Too

Compared to the best balance training in the world, T'ai Chi is about twice as effective. Some of the other balance exercises studied in the Ivy League study on balance were very expensive computer models that required participants to go into a lab and practice. The simple exercises of T'ai Chi are therefore not only much more effective than the other exercises, but they are very cheap.

You don't have to get a gym membership or an expensive physical trainer, or any fancy clothes or equipment. All you need are these terrific toys called your mind and your body. Now, *go play!*

T'ai Chi's Gentle to Arthritis and Your Joints

T'ai Chi is an exercise few doctors will ever tell patients to stop practicing. It provides perhaps the lowest impact weight-bearing exercise there is. We all need weight-bearing exercise to help build bone mass and connective tissue, but for those with rheumatoid arthritis or some other conditions weight-bearing exercise is a problem. For these people, weight-bearing exercise can aggravate joints, causing tenderness or swelling.

However, a study cited in the *American Journal of Physical Medicine and Rehabilitation* wanted to see if T'ai Chi would harm rheumatoid arthritis patients. To their pleasant surprise, T'ai Chi did no damage whatsoever and provided them with the safe weight-bearing exercise they seriously needed. The forms were modified for these patients, and everyone with arthritis or knee problems should be sure they only do forms that feel good to them. But this T'ai Chi discovery is good news for all of us because it gives us all a weight-bearing exercise that is safe even into old age.

T'ai Chi: the Health Care of the Future

Most Chinese hospitals have long integrated Western crisis medicine with Traditional Chinese Medicine. This is now rapidly happening in the United States as well. The American Medical Association recently recognized acupuncture as a valid treatment, which is causing Western doctors to look at T'ai Chi and QiGong even more intently.

Growing numbers of neurologists, cardiologists, general practitioners, physical therapists, hypertension specialists, and psychologists are already prescribing T'ai Chi and/or QiGong as treatment, or as supplemental treatment, for many conditions. In Part 6 you will find T'ai Chi prescribed for specific conditions.

As more Western scientific research is completed on the benefits of T'ai Chi and QiGong, this trend will expand, and we all will benefit greatly by lower health care costs.

T'ai Chi & QiGong's Healing Powers

When you first hear of the benefits of T'ai Chi and QiGong, it may sound like snake oil. This is because it is effective for helping to treat all things on all levels. "How can it do that?" you may ask. It does this by connecting us to the most powerful healing tool there is—the healing power of the mind. It is the power of the mind that is at the heart of our healing.

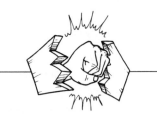

A T'ai Chi Punch Line

Studies have shown that if patients "believe" that something can cure them, the possibility that it will is much higher. Cynicism is found to be one of the single most hazardous behaviors for our health. I always tell students, "If I have a choice between being smart enough to realize I'm incurable, or stupid enough to fool myself into curing myself—I'll be the fool any day."

It is estimated that placebos can positively treat about 60 percent of our health problems. Placebos are sugar pills (or fake treatments) doctors sometimes give to fool patients into curing themselves. This gets the mind/body to trigger its own internal healing processes, by the mind simply telling itself it's OK for the body to heal. This indicates that the body has a tremendous potential to SELF HEAL, *if we believe in the cure.*

T'ai Chi and QiGong are not placebos. They are powerful health tools that can give us access to the tremendous natural healing power of the body, the power behind the placebo. Many of these healing benefits are documented, and new research is emerging all the time. It's important for you to understand just how powerful these tools are so that your mind will allow them to do their magic.

The Least You need to Know

➤ T'ai Chi facilitates the flow of Qi and health to your cells.

➤ Narrow thinking squeezes off life energy.

➤ T'ai Chi integrates the mind, body, and emotions.

➤ By toning our Qi, we tone all our healing systems.

➤ Only T'ai Chi provides an acupressure treatment and organ massage, while promoting circulation and centeredness.

➤ You don't have to memorize how it works, just relax and do it.

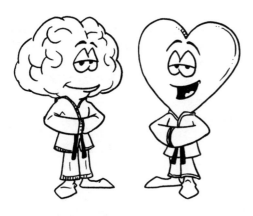

Chapter 4

T'ai Chi Expands the Mind and Lightens the Heart

In This Chapter

➤ Healing mentally and emotionally with T'ai Chi

➤ Discover the power of calm and peace

➤ The Unbendable Arm

➤ T'ai Chi reminds you that you are perfect

➤ Flexing your imagination muscle

The problem with the rat race is, even if you win the race, you're still a rat.

—Lily Tomlin

Our mental and emotional well-being is ravaged by the demands of the day-to-day rat race. T'ai Chi is not only a great physical workout and health tool, but can heal us mentally and emotionally by changing the way we look at life. T'ai Chi shows us that life does not have to be that hard.

The simple ways T'ai Chi and QiGong look at movement and life can be powerful self-improvement tools, as well as a soothing balm to our frazzled nerves.

T'ai Chi Calms the Rat Race, Healing Heart and Mind

Chinese masters constantly repeat, "Soong Yi-Dien" (loosen up). This instruction is not just to encourage a physical loosening, but a mental, emotional, and social loosening as well. The goal of T'ai Chi is to weave silken threads of calm into our lives, soothing us as we face the daily rat race. The calmer we are, the calmer our workplace and our home are.

However, at first, rather than bringing T'ai Chi's calm to the rat race, students often unconsciously bring the rat race into the T'ai Chi class or into their T'ai Chi practice at home. They do this because they want to "efficiently" learn T'ai Chi. Our work, lives, and technology are all geared towards making things happen faster and faster. So, we naturally want to "hurry up and relax." This can't happen. We have to let go of urgency and efficiency in order to truly and deeply experience what T'ai Chi offers. However, much to the surprise of many T'ai Chi students (including me), we soon realize that as T'ai Chi helps us become less urgent, we actually become more efficient. If this sounds impossible, read on.

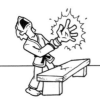

Ouch!

Many Western students feel hopeless upon learning that T'ai Chi is a lifelong process. We in the West are conditioned to expect immediate, short term results. Don't be discouraged. T'ai Chi is the lifelong process that gives immediate results. Even if you just took one T'ai Chi class and practiced what you learned, you would get great benefit. It just gets better and better for the rest of your life.

Frantic Action vs. Efficiency

T'ai Chi's ability to calm, energize, heal, strengthen, and tone the mind and body in a short half-hour workout is unequaled. However, if we try to do T'ai Chi efficiently, it doesn't work as well. It's when we relax and don't try that T'ai Chi works its magic.

The idea that we can get something very worthwhile done without being in high anxiety to hurry up and do it is a new concept for most of us.

T'ai Chi Is Smelling the Roses

Our heart and mind seem to be in a constant state of turmoil. With the tidal wave of information the information age has swept into our lives, we always feel two steps behind the pack. We struggle to understand the latest technology, knowing full well that a newer version will be out before we learn the one that just came out.

We forget to breathe and enjoy the *learning* in life, which is pretty much all there is to life when you get down to it. We are not and never will be done learning. So, we might as well smell the roses on the way.

Learning to "love the learning" of T'ai Chi is one of the most important lessons T'ai Chi offers our frantic lives. In T'ai Chi classes students sometimes come in gung-ho to learn one set of forms and move on. The concept that T'ai Chi is a lifelong process comes as a big shock. Students think they can hurry in, get fixed, get calmed, get healthy, and then get going. They want to hurry up and *finish,* so they can hurry up to finish the next thing they want to hurry up and do. But by living this way, our lives just become a lot of hurrying. There is no finish in T'ai Chi or life.

T'ai Chi's calming effects can be felt immediately the very first day of practice, but not if you hurry up to feel them. You have to let go of outcome and let the nice feelings be a pleasant surprise, rather than an urgent demand.

T'ai Chi's movements flow one into the other, just as life's events do. By learning how to breathe and relax the body, while moving through these events, we become an island of soothing calm even when in the center of the rat race. Our habit of letting the frantic demands of the day fill our mind becomes easier and easier to let go of as we practice T'ai Chi.

Remember to Breathe and Everything Else Takes Care of Itself

The very first thing students do in T'ai Chi class is to close their eyes and breathe. Take deep breaths all the way into the bottom of the lungs and then let go of the breath, the muscles, and the day. Let go of everything you've done before getting there and everything you plan to do later. Just be here and now, breathing.

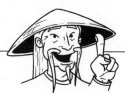

Sage Sifu Says

Go ahead—take a deep breath right now! Don't wait until you are in a quiet retreat or on the top of a mountain to use your T'ai Chi tools. Begin to weave the ideas of effortless breathing release into everything you do. If you remember to breathe, everything else will most likely take care of itself.

As your mind fills with remembering to breathe through your T'ai Chi movements and gravity forces you to focus on your balance, you must let go of the worries of the day.

You cannot do T'ai Chi without letting go of thoughts about what to defrost for dinner or the laundry that needs to be done.

T'ai Chi does not advocate starvation or wearing dirty clothes. It does, however, advocate being one hundred percent in the moment, whether its doing T'ai Chi or washing clothes. This is what is called mindfulness, or being here and now. You'll find that the more you can let go of the dinner and the laundry, to feel your breath, your muscles releasing, and the silken flow of your T'ai Chi movements, the more you'll enjoy doing the laundry or cooking dinner when you do get to it. The T'ai Chi practice of being here and now will seep into your daily life by reminding you to breathe as you move. As you do the laundry, you'll slow down and breathe, you'll feel the pleasure of the warmth of the clothes coming out of the dryer, and really enjoy the sweet scent of clean clothes. While making dinner, you'll relax and breathe, enabling you to truly smell the fragrance of dinner.

We don't have to race if we are always where we like being. Then we never have to fear looking in the mirror and seeing a racing rat.

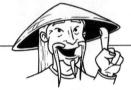

Sage Sifu Says

As T'ai Chi helps us "feel good" on a regular basis, we want more of that feeling. You may find yourself spending more time with people who nurture you and less time with those who put you down.

This is a powerfully healthful transformative part of doing T'ai Chi. As the movements in T'ai Chi teach you to ease around areas of discomfort in the body so as to expand mobility without injury, this echoes out into our lives. You begin to find nurturing ways to move and live socially.

The Power of Effortlessness

In our fast-paced dog-eat-dog world, it is hard to believe that we can be more powerful when we are not straining. However, that is exactly when we are most powerful, not only mentally and emotionally, *but also physically*. Because we are so conditioned to be mentally and emotionally straining all the time, many students feel "guilty" taking quiet still time to heal their minds and emotions from the strains of the day. Those students need a real physical example of how we function more effectively when relaxed. If you are a victim of this guilt, the following exercise will help you let your mind and emotions get the most out of T'ai Chi's effortless ways.

The Unbendable Arm

The unbendable arm is a terrific physical example of the concept of "effortless action" and how powerful that kind of action is. In the West we tend to think of big straining muscles and bursting head veins whenever we think of power.

T'ai Chi can rescue us from that sweaty, head-pounding delusion. In T'ai Chi, our goal is to move and stand with as little effort as possible. Ancient Taoist poets tried to explain in words the seemingly limitless power found in living lives of effortlessness with calm minds and quiet hearts. However, the concept of effortless power is so strange to Westerners that the following demonstration of the Unbendable Arm is worth a thousand words. (Note: If you have any arm or shoulder injuries, you may not want to do the Unbendable Arm exercise. Also, if you have difficulty performing it, you may want to practice the Sitting QiGong exercise in Part 3, and then try again.)

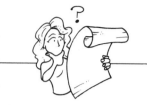

Know Your Chinese

The focus of **Taoist** (pronounced *dowist*) philosophy is the invisible force of nature's laws. When we are calm and still in our hearts, minds, and bodies, we can "feel" or "sense" the subtle direction of Tao. Living the Tao is the most effortless, meaningful way to live. In the West we may call the sense of the Tao a hunch or an intuition, or what feels right.

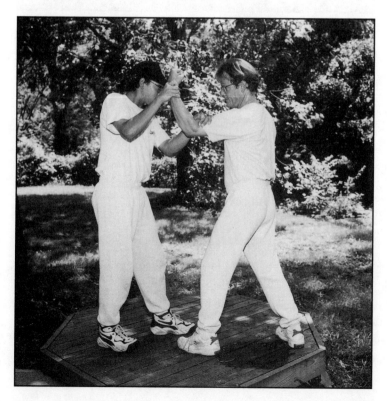

Notice the person is able to bend my arm even as I use all my muscular strength to resist.

However, notice here that my arm is relaxed, yet the larger person cannot bend it.

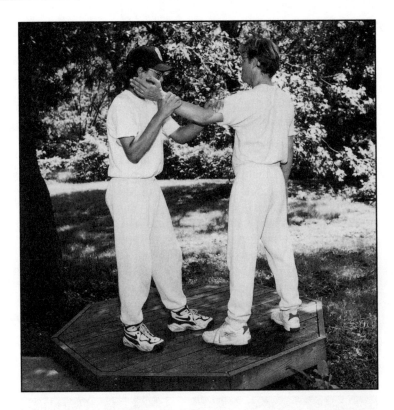

T'ai Sci

Taoist philosophy is a model used by many Western psychotherapists as they encourage patients to let go of obsessing on outcome and rather enjoying the "process" of life. In fact, T'ai Chi exercises are recommended as an active model to achieve these healing ends.

The Unbendable Arm is a powerful physical example of this principle of effortless power. In my class demonstrations I will ask the largest, most powerful-looking student to try to bend my arm. Resisting with all my muscular strength, they nevertheless eventually bend my arm. However, when I completely relax my mind and body, thinking of an empty flow, or of airy relaxation pouring through my head, shoulder, arm, and on out my fingers through the walls of the building, they can't bend it. The students strain to bend my relaxed arm, yet find they cannot.

Our Flexibility Is Our Strength

This Taoist principle of effortless power is even more meaningful in our mental and emotional lives.

I use the Unbendable Arm not to demonstrate the physical power of effortless motion (although it does demonstrate that), but to dispel the myth that our straining is equivalent to productivity. The Chinese say the most powerful T'ai Chi is like a supple bamboo, flexible and bendable, because obviously a rigid stick can be easily broken. Just as we relax our arms to make them strong, we can relax our minds to become more effective in life. We can relax our hearts and experience more profound and meaningful feelings. When we breathe and relax while typing at the keyboard or answering the phone, we are so much more effective and real. We have time for the people in our lives, instead of always rushing past them to get to the next urgent task.

Patterns vs. Chaos

T'ai Chi helps our bodies be more effective by relaxing the muscles. This allows a more ordered pattern of muscle use, so that muscles aren't fighting other muscles. Well, T'ai Chi has the same effect on the mind. By quieting the mind of all the daily "noise," our mind can open to more orderly patterns of thought.

Coaching the Mind Team

The way that the body fights itself physically with muscle tension, the mind also keeps itself in needless chaos with the noisy thoughts spinning around in it. T'ai Chi and QiGong can end this internal battle and enhance the power of the mind and imagination. Just as the slow deliberate motions of T'ai Chi calm the body and get the muscles to work together more powerfully (as demonstrated by the Unbendable Arm), that same calmness gets the mind to organize.

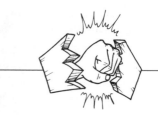

A T'ai Chi Punch Line

When studying T'ai Chi in Hong Kong as a young man, I was intrigued by the construction workers there. At the time I was in great shape, being a karate enthusiast who trained very hard. However, I was humbled by the much smaller thinner Chinese construction workers hauling enormously heavy bags of cement up bamboo scaffolds on their thin shoulders. They showed barely any exertion. Whether the workers practiced T'ai Chi or not, they had obviously absorbed some of its principles.

Imagine that life is like a football game, and we keep getting batted around by really big linemen that we call problems. The noise in our heads is deafening, as every time we get up from being knocked down, another big problem bangs into us. Its hard to even think about solutions when big problems bang into us one after another.

Now, imagine that we could somehow be lifted up above the chaos to look down on what's happening from a higher, clearer angle, like a coach in the upper deck of the stadium. We would see patterns, or plays, forming. We would see how waves of linemen or problems flow. We could make adjustments before problems are right in our face, enabling us to choose the path of least resistance, not only making it easier, but getting much more yardage with each play. T'ai Chi practice continually lifts our mind to that higher clearer perception.

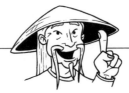

Sage Sifu Says

The Taoist philosophers took a holistic approach to the world, meaning that they saw each little thing as kind of a model for bigger structures. For example, each cell in our body makes up the whole body, as individuals we make up our family, our family makes the neighborhood, which makes the city, state, and society. Therefore, the most powerful contribution we can make to the world is to be the healthiest we can be, physically, mentally and emotionally. If our health heals the world around us, then a healthier world around us also heals us. This is the kind of cycle that needs to spin out of control.

Innercise Integrates Outer Relationships

Phil Jackson, former head coach of the World Champion Chicago Bulls, is a Zen practitioner, and he introduced the entire Chicago Bulls team to Zen exercises.

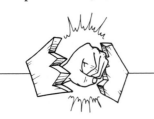

A T'ai Chi Punch Line

The Chinese Character for Qi, or life energy, and the Latin root spir, as in spirit, means the air we breathe. Both ancient cultures obviously saw how our breath connects us to the life force. When considering that each of us has breathed an atom of oxygen that was breathed by Jesus, Buddha, and Mohammed, the Taoist claim that we are all connected becomes a very real concept.

T'ai Chi and QiGong exercises are from the same roots as Zen exercises and are often indistinguishable from them.

The year that the Bulls were introduced to Zen practices, was the year that they became the winningest team in the history of the NBA. This is no coincidence. The choreography displayed by the Bulls that year was mind boggling; the team often resembled one living entity, rather than five different players. As Zen exercise allows the mind to clear itself of its daily chatter or rubble, it also clarifies the communication between people. So, just as the Bulls players began to quiet and clarify their own internal function by relaxing muscles and quieting thoughts they didn't need, they simultaneously clarified their player-to-player communication. This clarity is what we saw in the incredible plays the Bulls made that year.

This same clarity we cultivate through our daily T'ai Chi or QiGong exercises can help us clarify our relationships with others at work or home. Most social breakdowns are rooted in a lack of clarity, for if we aren't clear on what we want and need, we can never expect others to support our efforts. Whether its our love life, our family, our work, or social relationships, T'ai Chi's soothing way of moving through life will make relationships more healing and effortless.

People around us become easier to deal with when we are easier to deal with. T'ai Chi shows us how much of the external world reflects what goes on in our own heart and mind. Dressage, the national magazine for the Olympic horseback riding style, promotes T'ai Chi as perhaps the most effective exercise a rider can perform to enhance riding skills. What's fascinating is why.

The article said that horses pick up on the riders mental and emotional stress levels. Therefore, if the rider does T'ai Chi before mounting his horse, the horse gives a smoother and quicker ride.

Imagine how much your unconscious mental and emotional turmoil affects those around you at home or work. Then think of how much your life would change if you did T'ai Chi before riding in.

T'ai Chi-hut-hut-BREAK from Old Patterns

This is what T'ai Chi and QiGong can do. T'ai Chi's physical model of moving with the muscles relaxing off of the bones is a model for letting go of mental and emotional obsessions. T'ai Chi allows us let go of the chaos of life and lets our minds lift and observe, unattached to outcomes, grudges, or obsessive desires. It allows us to see more clearly the patterns that cause us to bump our head into the same old walls again and again.

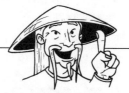

Sage Sifu Says

The life force is clarity and simplicity and holds no need to compete.
By letting go of desires, utmost calm is realized, and all the world arrives at effortless peace.

Letting go of attachments or stepping out of the game from time to time gives us a fresh perspective. Fresh perspective is what allows us to exercise our "imagination muscle." It's the most effortless thing you can do. However, it's not always easy because it requires you to let go of all your thoughts, plans, and regrets. Creating space or breathing room in our busy days with T'ai Chi and QiGong helps our minds to let go of old patterns. This allows our mind to open to the pure inspiration that wants to bubble up inside it.

T'ai Chi Dispels the Idea of Wrongness

The most mentally and emotionally healing concept T'ai Chi has to offer our hypercritical world may be that T'ai Chi dispels the idea of "wrongness." When you practice T'ai Chi, you never ever do it "wrong." You just do it. Each time you do it, you relax a little more, you breathe a little easier, and your T'ai Chi gets a little better.

Ouch!

If you study with a T'ai Chi instructor who is hypercritical, you may want to find another one who has more fun with T'ai Chi. However, be aware that if you are hypercritical of yourself by nature, you may unconsciously project that onto the instructor. Relax and enjoy yourself when in T'ai Chi class and when practicing at home. This will help your instructor relax too.

T'ai Chi is a Model for Life

The effortless sustenance T'ai Chi offers our lives is the understanding that we are always "perfect," That our lives are ever evolving perfection. When we learn things about T'ai Chi that we can improve, it is much easier to adopt the new ways if the old ways don't have to be "wrong." This is one of the ways T'ai Chi makes a terrific model for life in general.

Our culture's concepts of wrongness constipate the ability to let go of old ways and move into new ways more easily. If something must be wrong before it can be discarded, we judge ourselves as wrong for having done it that way. If we see things in an ever-evolving state of improvement, then nothing is wrong, and there are always better ways. Then we can see that we were right for having done it the old way, but can be even "righter" for doing it a new way.

The only wrong thing you can do in T'ai Chi is to tell yourself you're wrong.

T'ai Chi Breaks Limits

T'ai Chi's way of seeing exercise (and life) as a process leaves us always content with where we are, while always taking us past our old limits. When we obsess over getting things "right," whether we know it or not, we limit ourselves by thinking we are "done" when we get it "right." By giving up that myth, we begin to feel a limitlessness to life. T'ai Chi helps us feel bigger, dream bigger, and love bigger.

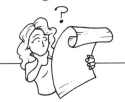

Know Your Chinese

The character for **Qi** (pronounced chee) represents steam rising from rice, meaning the air of life, a symbol for effortless sustenance.

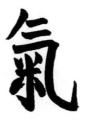

Qi

Notice that the Qi character is a combination of steam or air (the top half) and rice (the lower half).

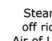

Steam rising off rice is the Air of Life, *or Qi*

Steam rising off rice

Rice

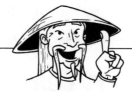

Sage Sifu Says

"When problems arise, use your energy to fix the problem, rather than wasting energy fixing the blame. Fix the problem, not the blame." This concept goes right to the heart of what T'ai Chi offers our harried lives.

Each time you do T'ai Chi, you relax a little more deeply and become a little more self-aware, enabling you to continually improve your T'ai Chi.

When we stick with T'ai Chi long enough, we realize that our T'ai Chi improves each time we do it. More importantly it helps us see that we never did T'ai Chi "wrong," for T'ai Chi is not a destination where a fixed level of perfection exists. Like our lives, T'ai Chi is an unfolding rose of improvement that blooms endlessly, more perfectly, and more beautifully each new day that we practice it.

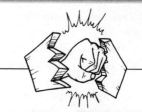

A T'ai Chi Punch Line

An 80-year old T'ai Chi teacher was being interviewed about his 60 years of T'ai Chi practice. The interviewer asked him, "At what point did you feel you mastered T'ai Chi?"

The old teacher replied, "I'll let you know as soon as I do."

T'ai Chi Enhances Life

Does T'ai Chi make life perfect? No, not more perfect than it already is. And it is always perfect, although sometimes it may seem perfectly miserable. T'ai Chi encourages us to let go of outcomes, and simply pour our energy into whatever nourishes life, our life, and all life. The flow of Qi through the body is like water through the roots of a plant. It doesn't fix anything in particular, it just enhances life.

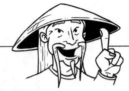

Sage Sifu Says

The best people are like water. Water nurtures all things and never is in competition with them.

—Lao Tzu, Taoist philosopher, sixth century B.C.

T'ai Sci

The *alpha state* is a frequency of brain waves that occurs during a state of relaxed concentration. It is one of four brain wave frequencies: delta is the slowest, prevalent during infancy or in adults during sleep; theta is present in drowsy barely conscious states; alpha, during QiGong relaxation exercises; and beta is common when the mind is busy or restless.

T'ai Chi and QiGong Strengthen the Imagination Muscle

Sitting QiGong is a motionless exercise. So, if the slowness of T'ai Chi makes it seem ineffective to many Westerners, the stillness of QiGong may seem like a colossal waste of time. However, this could not be farther from the truth.

These slow mindful exercises bring the brain into a very calm state known by scientists as the alpha state. This is a highly creative state of mind. In fact three of the great discoverers of our time had their greatest insights while in alpha states. Albert Einstein, Thomas Edison, and Nikolai Tesla all claimed to get their greatest discoveries while in a state of mind that Einstein called "wakeful rest."

Alpha States Expand Your Mind

Why is the alpha state such a creative state of mind? There are two reasons. One is that when our mind is filled with normal daily worries, plans, and television/radio noise, there is no room for creative thought. Two, there may be a deeper knowledge within our minds that we can't access when our minds are busy with daily problem solving. The psychologist Carl Jung said there is a "collective unconscious" that holds great knowledge, and that we all have access to it. But when our mind is busy with balancing the checkbook or worrying about our next raise, we can't open up to that great knowledge. This collective unconscious is the ocean of information our minds get ideas from. It is like all the info on the Internet, and our minds are like the computers that can download that information.

QiGong Expands Our Minds

When we are tense, our minds are tight and closed to new ideas. This resembles the problem we now have with the Internet. The Internet has loads of great information, but most of our computers seem to take forever to get to it. This is because information bottlenecks when it passes through the system's modems because these modems have a limited bandwidth. If your brain is like your computer, and ideas are like the Internet, then QiGong and T'ai Chi are a way to increase that bandwidth to allow much more access to information.

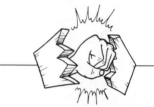

A T'ai Chi Punch Line

Bet ya your brain's in beta! The stress we feel in our busy lives is partly because our mind spends too much time in beta brain waves, or "busy brain waves." QiGong can help you drop into a calm state even when you're in line at the supermarket.

We've all experienced this whether you know it or not. Have you ever faced a really tough problem that you couldn't solve. No matter how hard you tried, you couldn't see the solution. Then when you gave up, and went for a walk, or sat on the back porch, or went for a drive, the answer came to you. You saw a pattern you missed when your mind was too busy trying to put pieces together. Then when you gave up, your mind put the pieces together very easily and very effectively.

This is what T'ai Chi and QiGong help us learn to do more often and more easily. They open our mental bandwidth by allowing the mind to let go of its clutter. Things get clearer. So, Einstein, now you can see that T'ai Chi and QiGong are far from a waste of time.

The Least You Need to Know

➤ T'ai Chi heals your mind and heart.

➤ Real power comes from peace of mind.

➤ T'ai Chi teaches that life is limitless.

➤ Stress closes the mind, but QiGong opens it.

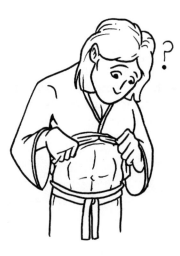

The Spirit of T'ai Chi Is Finding Our Center

> **In This Chapter**
>
> ➤ Being here and now
>
> ➤ Letting go of the fight or flight response
>
> ➤ Kicking our adrenaline addiction
>
> ➤ What is a master? *You are!*
>
> ➤ Using T'ai Chi to change your world

Usually we don't think about being in or out of "center" until life is completely out of hand. Then we know we are out of it, but we're still not sure what *it* is that we're out of. We often think we are just out of our minds.

Chapter 5 can make you an expert on what the center is. Then all you need to do is practice the QiGong exercises in Part 3 and the T'ai Chi in Part 4 and 5 to feel how good the center feels when you're in it. Being in center reduces the melodrama in your life, so you can focus more attention on the big stuff.

Standing in the center means aligning our physical, emotional, mental, and spiritual selves so that we function at our very best, using everything we've got in everything we do. This centering capability of T'ai Chi may seem spiritual, but it is really a kind of science that understands that our mind, body, emotions, and spirit are all intertwined, and that if we integrate them through T'ai Chi practice, we become more powerful. If our body and mind work together to nurture our emotional and spiritual well-being rather than against each other as they sometimes do, life may be less dramatic but much more fulfilling.

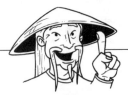

Sage Sifu Says

A wonderful American interpretation of Zen philosophy is, "No matter where ya go, there ya are." All the toys, trips, and movies in the world cannot take you away from yourself. T'ai Chi is about being right in the center of where you are right now, rather than running from it.

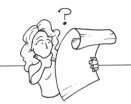

Know Your Chinese

The word **Zen** is a Japanese translation of the Chinese word *ch'an*. Both are translations of the original Sanskrit word *dhyana* (pronounced *jyana*). They describe an art often called "just sitting," or *za-zen*. While one sits in Zen meditation, the mind does not calculate or figure, but is still and calm within, like a glass of muddy water slowly becoming clear as it sits still.

T'ai Chi-ing Zen and Now

T'ai Chi helps us stand right in the center of our lives by focusing the mind and body to release stress that blocks awareness of our spiritual nature and needs.

Often, it seems like life is a merry-go-round, and we're hanging on by our last fingernail as the demands of life pull at us with everything they've got. This is what being "out of center" refers to. When we are out there on the edge just trying to survive, we are not very creative. In fact, we often complicate our lives even more with various coping behaviors. Some cope by over-charging their credit cards on compulsive spending. Others smoke compulsively or turn to alcohol or drugs. Still others become adrenaline junkies who can't slow down and have to be doing something all the time. All of these behaviors have one thing in common; they all distract us from the turmoil going on inside our own minds and hearts. T'ai Chi is like a Zen exercise. Zen is an art of *being still*, not running from problems, but being here and now.

T'ai Chi slows us down inside and out. As our bodies begin to move more slowly, our breathing slows down. As we hear our breathing slow, our mind begins to ride on the rhythm of that relaxed breath, letting go bit by bit of the storming thoughts of the day. As the mind calms it has a resonant effect on the heartbeat, the blood pressure, and the healing systems of the body. On some level we begin to realize we are not in a state of mortal danger after all, which is a state that our ancient "fight or flight" response produces in us. It is this response more than the world around us that makes life seem like it is spinning way out of control.

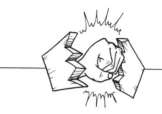

A T'ai Chi Punch Line

Lao Tzu (pronounced *low*, as in "OW!", *dzoo*) wrote, "In doing nothing, all things are done." He wasn't advocating laziness. He meant that by breathing, relaxing, and enjoying whatever it is that we do, all things get done, yet seem so effortless that we feel like we did nothing.

Fight or Flight—or T'ai Chi

Feeling panicked by life is something we all experience much more often than we want to think about. This feeling is a product of the reflex response called the *fight or flight response*. This reflex response is like an old memory held in the cells of our body, a cellular memory from our caveman (or cavewoman) days, when we were the grade A prime rib for saber-toothed tigers. We automatically respond to stress by breathing shallowly and tightening every muscle in our bodies so as not to be heard and to be ready to run like heck or bash the head of our would-be-diner.

T'ai Chi Bring Caveman to Modern World, Ugh!

Our modern problem is this. Our cells still think they live in a prehistoric world where mortal danger is everywhere. Our outdated response to stress often leaves us in a minor (or not so minor) panic at every red light, supermarket line, or computer glitch we encounter.

This response worked well back then because we really didn't have many options. It does not, however, serve us very well today. Although sometimes the thought of either attacking the source of our anxiety or running away from it seems mighty appealing, it doesn't bode well for our next job performance review.

ROOM FOR IMPROVEMENT: Bill should attempt to attack fewer coworkers this quarter, and an emphasis on not fleeing from customers is highly recommended.

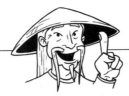

Sage Sifu Says

The natural breathing that T'ai Chi and QiGong promote is a powerful antidote to the fight or flight response. Just remembering to breathe when crisis hits can significantly affect your ability to better handle it.

T'ai Chi Stops the Fight and Slows the Flight

On a cellular level the fight or flight response is just as inappropriate. When we go into that mode, our heart pounds, our blood pressure elevates, oxygen consumption increases, and blood lactate levels (anxiety levels) increase. If it happens often enough, it can actually cause our brain to shrink.

When we enter this state, the energy flowing through our bodies becomes very erratic, like a stormy sea. When we practice our T'ai Chi and things begin to calm and center, our energy begins to flow more smoothly and evenly. The Chinese call this "smooth Qi." Smooth Qi is a healthful state produced by doing T'ai Chi. It soothes our bodies and begins to sooth our minds as well. Some would say T'ai Chi actually starts calming the mind, and then the body becomes calm. Either way it is a pretty helpful thing to be able to do.

T'ai Sci

Studies show that about 80 percent of illness is due to stress, and that the six leading causes of death are stress related. Most stress-related damage is caused by adrenaline addiction. According to these studies, most of our illnesses are self-inflicted, which means that we are creating our own health care crisis. T'ai Chi could help us to break our adrenaline addiction, while also helping to dramatically lower health care and insurance costs in the long run.

Withdrawal from Adrenaline

Many of us have actually become addicted to the feeling of anxiety, just like a cigarette smoker gets addicted to the energy level nicotine doses provide. So, at first T'ai Chi or QiGong may cause you to feel drained.

If this happens, hang in there. You are going through an adrenaline withdrawal. As you continue to practice your T'ai Chi and QiGong, you will eventually break through that wall of drowsiness and boredom. You will discover that you can have the best of both worlds. You will experience the relaxed energy that T'ai Chi creates in you as you find your center.

As the flow of Qi opens up throughout your mind and body, you will have limitless energy, but without the edge. You will run with plenty of juice, but be attuned to when it's time to rest, and you will be able to rest when its time. You'll feel less and less need to be endlessly busy all the time, but you'll have limitless energy for the truly important things in your life. Furthermore, the calmness that T'ai Chi fosters will grant you the wisdom to know what activities are important and which are not.

Today is a good day to get off adrenaline and get to the real juice. Breathe, breathe some more, and do T'ai Chi.

A T'ai Chi Master: What Is That?

T'ai Chi and martial arts abound with myths of super human feats performed by masters who defy physical reality. These feats may be true. Some masters have been known to break bricks with their heads. Although, having never been attacked by a brick, I'm not sure what the point is. I'm usually only attacked by stress, fear, and anxiety.

Actually, these performances are powerful demonstrations of the power of internal effortlessness and focus. Often, however, these bizarre demonstrations are a distraction from the real point of these wonderful tools. What T'ai Chi and QiGong offer us is much more miraculous than the ability to break bricks; they help us understand ourselves and how we fit into the world. They make us masters of our own destiny instead of victims of circumstance. Of course, real masters understand that we are never in control, but merely copilots of our destiny. However, a copilot is preferable to and more powerful than being an unwitting passenger on this first class ride we call life.

Manifest (Physical) vs. Unmanifest (Energy)

Does it seem like life is one surprise after another? Look again. Our physical bodies are the manifest part of who we are. Our thoughts are the unmanifest part of us that creates our bodies. So, our bodies are like reflections of our mind. Our thoughts are energy that triggers feelings or emotions and that actually changes our physical body. These emotions turn the energy of thoughts into physical responses, just as chronic worry can create ulcers.

Consider this: Remember when Old Yeller died at the end of the movie? It broke your heart and made you cry, didn't it? *Come on, you know it did.* Well, the thought about Old Yeller dying at the end of the movie caused a deep emotional swell; our eyes water, and it actually feels like our heart is about to break. So, thoughts change our bodies

T'ai Sci

Centuries ago, Chinese Taoist philosophers wrote that all things are formed from the same field of potential energy. As modern physics explains it, all atomic particles emerge from the same energy field, meaning that all things in the universe are made of the same essential energy. We are all therefore connected to everything else, to each other, and to the universe.

through the communication of emotions. Put simply, our mind in some ways creates our bodies.

One of the fascinating things QiGong shows us is that the thoughts we are aware of are actually just reflections of what goes on inside us on even deeper levels. Most of our consciousness is subconscious, or below the surface of our awareness. Our thoughts and emotions, and lastly our physical bodies, are results or reflections of an even deeper part of us. That deeper part is the unmanifest part of ourselves. QiGong and T'ai Chi's ability to connect us to that deeper, unmanifest part of ourselves is a powerful self-improvement tool.

Imagine that our lives are like a big fountain drink glass of 7 Up. If you stand up and look down into it, you only see the bubbles bursting up into the air from the surface. This represents the manifest, or obvious, part of life. From this angle you don't see the deep liquid below that formed these bubbles.

As we experience events in our lives, we are only seeing the bubbles popping up from the surface and not what formed them. These emerging bubbles may take the form of successes, or reoccurring problems. Perhaps we go from one bad relationship to another or constantly fight with our kids.

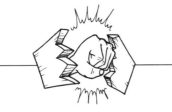

A T'ai Chi Punch Line

Lao Tzu, the foremost Taoist philosopher, wrote, "the sage puts himself last and finds himself in the foremost place." Modern research shows that those who volunteer or lead lives of service to others are usually far healthier than those who do not.

However, T'ai Chi, and especially QiGong, meditation let us sit down and look at the "7 Up glass of life" from the side, allowing us to see the source of the bubbles. Here we can see that those bubbles, or events of our lives, actually form way down below the surface. This being the unmanifest, or unconscious, part of life.

So our quiet meditations place us sitting on the side observing the true depth of life. Here we see experiences are really end results, rather than big surprises. Events in our lives are actually results of patterns or habits we have below the level of what we usually see and feel. We set ourselves up for success or failure by how we think of ourselves every day. If we think of ourselves as valuable human beings, capable of success, then we're much more likely to form bubbles that pop on the surface of our lives in the form of success stories.

Likewise, if we continually think of ourselves as bad or worthless, we will probably form bubbles to reflect that worthlessness in the form of relationship problems. Because if we believe that we are worthless, then we will attract people into our lives who will reinforce that reality. "Pop, pop, pop." Seeing only the pops makes us feel like victims of life.

Masters Are No Longer Victims

Being a T'ai Chi or QiGong master means we are no longer content to remain ignorant of the unmanifest part of life.

However, it's not enough just to know that our responses and actions in life have deeper roots. We have to find ways to change the patterns that form those bubbles way down below the surface of our lives. T'ai Chi and QiGong can help do this. By quieting our mind and body, they can allow us to feel inside where we hurt or hate. By feeling the source inside, we can begin to let it go. For example, if we have a grudge or unresolved hatred in our heart, we may walk around with a chip on our shoulder. The world will quickly give us confirmation for our grudge or hatred because people we meet will seem cold to us as we greet everyone with the chip on our shoulder, which makes us seem cold to them.

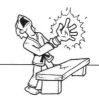

Ouch!

Modern psychology says that we are bombarded on many levels by information and stress that we never consciously perceive. Therefore, trying to attach mental reasons to feelings of being out of control, frightened, or stressed, is often a futile exercise. T'ai Chi helps us let go of stress on deep levels that we will never even notice.

Another example is sometimes I get angry with my kids, but what I'm actually responding to are things I hold inside. When I realize this, my responses change. I find that practicing my quiet T'ai Chi or QiGong meditation when I get home allows me to be clearer with my kids. I clear out stuff inside, so that if I do have a problem with their blasting stereo or whatever, I am responding to that and not to something I brought home from the office (or from my childhood). By being more aware of the dynamic of our lives, we feel less like victims. We can begin to affect our world more clearly.

As our lives become less cluttered with bubbles of discord, there is more room for a limitlessly flowing geyser of life energy or Qi to course through us. We become a geyser watering and nurturing everyone and everything lucky enough to be around us.

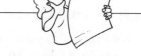

Know Your Chinese

The **I-Ching** (pronounced *ee-ching*), also known as *The Book of Changes,* is an ancient Chinese book of divination. This book is used to tell fortunes or to advise people on life decisions.

T'ai Chi and QiGong's daily pattern of reminding ourselves that we can *change* with ease, and feel safe in the world without constant muscle-tensing apprehension is a powerful tool. Sometimes it seems as though the body literally squeezes past burdens within each and every cell. T'ai Chi's ability to allow the body to release those burdens held from the past so each cell can fill with and be nurtured by life energy is a powerful way to affirm that we are worthy of success and love. On levels deeper than we can ever understand, T'ai Chi's easy and pleasant tools help create bubbles in the deepest part of our hearts and minds that burst outward and upward in lives that reflect our very best potential. Cheers, Master! Yeah, that's you.

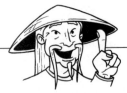

Sage Sifu Says

The Kuang Ping Yang Style of T'ai Chi is a series of 64 integrated postures, one changing always into the other. The 64 postures symbolize the 64 possibilities of *change* represented in the *I-Ching*. The essence of the I-Ching is that life is a constant flow of changing circumstances. Its lesson is that we cannot find security by holding onto any one thing or way of being, but by learning to *change* easily and smoothly as life dictates we must.

Master Your Own Self

As discussed earlier, the six leading causes of death are stress related. Since stress is something that we *can* control by practicing T'ai Chi and QiGong, using these tools means that we can powerfully affect our future in a positive way.

Luck of the Draw

We all are born with natural tendencies to height or weight, or, for some, diabetes or heart disease. Our genes give us those tendencies. However, we can play a big role in how those genes play out. If we drink or smoke heavily and ignore a healthy diet, we can help increase the possibility of the onset of diabetes and heart disease, while likely stunting our growth in length and expanding our growth in width.

On the other hand, we have been lucky enough to live in an age when T'ai Chi is as available as Coca-Cola. We have the ability to put an eternal ace up our sleeve, which heavily stacks the odds in our favor to live long, healthy, productive lives.

Gut Feelings: Tuning Your T'ai Chi Antennae

My T'ai Chi classes for children always began with one simple question, "Can you feel the inside of your bodies?" With little hands pressing into tiny rib cages, their puzzled faces would usually answer no. My next question was, "Have you ever felt a stomach ache or a headache?" Obviously, they all had.

T'ai Chi and QiGong are about moving the body, but it is also about feeling the body from the inside. We can feel pain inside, so we can also feel pleasure, and awareness of these feelings enables us to detect normal or abnormal function at a very early stage. By becoming attuned to our internal function, by quieting down, moving slowly, and listening to the signals inside our body, we tune our T'ai Chi antennae. We become conscious of our heart beat and our respiration rate.

What amazes most people is that we can affect our heart rate and respiration rate by using some simple QiGong methods to becoming aware of them. This is only the beginning. In my children's T'ai Chi classes, I asked children how it felt when they got nervous in school or were in trouble. They described feelings of "tight shoulders," "tight hearts," "tight chests," "hard to breathe," and so on. I asked them to make themselves feel that way, having them squench their shoulders and tighten their chests. Then I asked them to take in a deep breath and to let their chest and shoulders relax like a cloud floating in the sky on the exhale. I asked them to close their eyes and repeat this until they could feel their shoulders and chest relaxing and expanding from the inside.

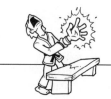

Ouch!

Dr. Andrew Weil, the Harvard educated medical doctor who now promotes Traditional Chinese Medical tools as part of his medical practice, claims shallow breathing is the main threat to our health. By becoming more conscious of our breath and breathing more fully, we may avoid the health problems many of our shallow breathing peers seem condemned to.

Try it. Pull your shoulders way up by your ears until your shoulders are very tight, and you can feel that tension. Tighten up all your head muscles as well, and feel that tension. Now, take a deep breath, close your eyes, and let go of everything as you release the breath; feel every cell of your body releasing that breath—absolute effortlessness, absolute letting go on a cellular level. Feel how good that release feels in the muscles in your shoulders and back, and how with every breath you let out, they relax a little more. Enjoy the tingling as blood and Qi flow back into those areas.

Our body is a playground of sensation. T'ai Chi exercises and QiGong methods are games we can play in that playground. It's fun, and it makes us healthy. What a deal!

T'ai Chi Can Affect the World Around Us

As you practice T'ai Chi daily, you begin to find that it has an affect on the world around you, not just the world inside your body. Shao Lin folklore spoke of T'ai Chi masters being invisible. What that may have referred to is the way their nonabrasive personalities allowed them to blend in unnoticed. For example, if two men walk into the same bar, one pushy and ill-tempered and the other very nonassuming, the bar will be more dangerous for the ill-tempered man.

What You See Is What You Get

In many ways we create the world we see by our expectations. If we push ourselves relentlessly, not taking time to enjoy life, we will likely see a hard driven merciless world around us. If we are cantankerous and mean, we will likely draw out those aspects of the people we meet. If we are filled with endless desires for things that we do not have, we will see a world of scarcity and desperation. Conversely, the man who is generally content with what he has will see a world of plenty. T'ai Chi is a celebration of our existence. It slows us down each day, long enough to remember how wonderful it is just to be able to move and breathe, live and feel. It nourishes our contentment. This makes us a healing force in our world, and a healthier world makes us a healthier person.

T'ai Chi and QiGong Are Inner-Space Suits

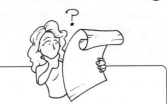

Know Your Chinese

Taoism (pronounced *dowism*) is an ancient Chinese philosophy of life. Its premise is that life flows through us and all living things the way ocean currents flow through the ocean. The Tao nurtures life and cannot be defined because it applies to all things. Taoists believe we should flow with the Tao, the way a surfer rides the waves, while adding our own flare and best intentions to its currents.

T'ai Chi and QiGong can help us focus our view of the world.

Look out your window. Do you see a tree, the sky, traffic, smog? Move your chair until all you see is the most pleasing aspect of what your window offers you. Each time you take a break from your work, resume this position and enjoy the view.

Our lives are our minds looking through a window at the world. At any given time we can see the best our world can be or the worst it can be. In fact, the state of our world has as much or perhaps even more to do with where *we are* as it does with where the world *is*. Two people can look at the same situation and see two entirely different things. For example, one person could look at a family and see a miracle they were blessed to be a part of, while another might look at the same situation and view it as a burden on his life, a prison he is sentenced to. In fact, even the same person may see his/her life as either of those things on any given day.

After seeing our world from space, Astronauts have experienced a dramatic change in the way they viewed life. They spoke of how precious life on Earth seemed from out there; even the things we think of as annoying, the arguments, and traffic seemed so precious from outer space.

By helping us to let go of our attachments to life's annoyances and allowing our minds to travel to "inner space," T'ai Chi and QiGong give us a view adjustment. We begin to notice that the things our children or coworkers do that are irritating are irritating because of the way we look at them. With T'ai Chi and QiGong, we get to pull back and remember how precious each moment is. What could be more helpful?

The Least You Need to Know

➤ T'ai Chi puts you in the center, right here and right now.

➤ T'ai Chi helps you cope with modern life without stress.

➤ T'ai Chi helps you think creatively.

➤ T'ai Chi changes the world, by changing your view of it.

Part 2
Suiting Up and Setting Out

After Part 1's explanation of the wonders of T'ai Chi, you are probably asking, "How do I sign up?" Part 2 will prepare you for your first T'ai Chi class, fashion wise and otherwise. However, for those with T'ai Chi experience, it may also provide valuable insights on how to make your ongoing T'ai Chi experience even more meaningful, both internally and externally.

Knowing when and where to do T'ai Chi can enrich your T'ai Chi experience and can even help treat certain health conditions. You will also learn the ins and outs of T'ai Chi etiquette and how to get the most out of T'ai Chi by becoming aware of the different ways it is taught.

Even advanced T'ai Chi students can benefit from Part 2's explanation of some of the mental and emotional challenges T'ai Chi practitioners encounter. For advanced students, you will find validation of your own experiences. For beginners, these insights will prepare you for those same challenges so that you can ride them out and hang in there for the long beautiful haul with T'ai Chi.

Part 2 will conclude by providing you with interesting and helpful T'ai Chi and martial arts terms, so that when you enter class you'll know what's being said. More importantly, Part 2 will enlighten you as to the deep and long-term goals of T'ai Chi exercises, enabling you to enjoy T'ai Chi's benefits right from the beginning.

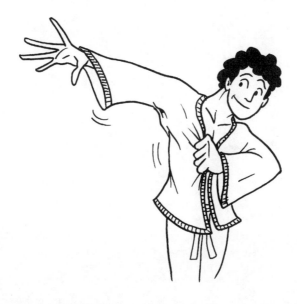

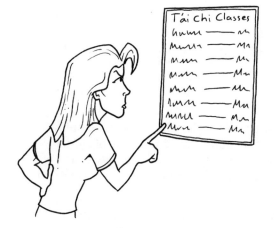

Finding the Right T'ai Chi Class

In This Chapter

➤ Where do I learn T'ai Chi?

➤ How much does T'ai Chi cost?

➤ How often do you do T'ai Chi?

➤ Choosing an instructor

➤ Choosing a style right for you

There are many ways to learn T'ai Chi. T'ai Chi's main lesson is to find the most "effortless" way to live. Therefore, you do not want to force yourself into a square hole, being the round peg that you are. You want to find the class that best suits you. Since everyone is different, T'ai Chi is perfect because T'ai Chi can be learned in many different ways.

Chapter 6 will help you decide what class is right for you, informing you of what's available and providing you with some questions to ask yourself. The more clear you are on what you want from T'ai Chi, the easier it will be for an instructor to fulfill those needs or to point you to another class that can.

Where Are Classes Held?

Just as T'ai Chi is good for so many different things, it is also offered in many different venues. What benefits you seek from T'ai Chi may help determine where you want to study T'ai Chi.

Business T'ai Chi for Employees

Many company Wellness Programs are beginning to offer T'ai Chi classes for employees. Ask your employer. Of course, you may want to study T'ai Chi outside of work or in addition to the company class. Don't limit yourself to taking only the classes at work (however, many company classes are subsidized, so this can be an incentive to do it at work).

If you take a work class and enjoy the instructor but would feel more comfortable with a class outside of work, ask the instructor about other classes he or she offers.

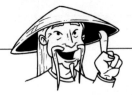

Sage Sifu Says

Try not to use only your head when choosing a T'ai Chi class. Just because the school looks nice, or the credentials sound great, or the instructor has studied for a gazillion years doesn't mean that it is the right school for you. When you talk with the instructor, how do you feel? That is the most important question.

Martial Arts Studios

Many of the "hard" martial arts studios specializing in karate, kung fu, or kenpo are beginning to offer T'ai Chi classes as well. In fact, a few have offered them for many years. Be aware, however, that martial arts studio classes will often focus on the martial applications of T'ai Chi.

Usually, these classes will be more comfortable to someone who is interested in a more athletically demanding form of T'ai Chi. These classes may involve a gentle sparing technique known as Push Hands, although Push Hands has many mental and emotional purposes as well.

Even if you are not interested in T'ai Chi's more athletic or martial applications, you should not rule out a martial arts studio until you speak with the instructor. Every instructor has their own style and where they teach may not necessarily indicate how they teach or what their focus is.

Senior Centers

Many community centers or senior centers offer T'ai Chi classes geared toward seniors. If you have a chronic condition that limits your mobility or are rehabilitating from an injury, you may find these classes very helpful. These classes generally progress at a slower, gentler rate than T'ai Chi for the general population.

Being a senior, however, doesn't mean that these are the classes you need. Many seniors want to learn more quickly, are up to more physical challenges, and may find they enjoy a general community class or even a martial arts studio class. You can't judge a T'ai Chi-er by his cover. In fact, the more you do T'ai Chi, the younger your "cover" is going to look.

T'ai Sci

Complications from falling injuries is the sixth largest cause of death among seniors. In a study done by Emory University, T'ai Chi was shown to be nearly twice as effective as any other balance conditioning exercise.

Community Center and Hospital Classes

Many cities' parks and recreation departments now offer T'ai Chi classes, as do many hospitals. These classes are usually for the general population and will include students of all ages. Generally, these classes will progress through learning movements at a little faster pace than the senior program classes do. However, even the briskest pace is usually quite manageable if you spend a little time each day practicing between your weekly or semi-weekly classes.

Church Classes

Many houses of worship now offer T'ai Chi classes. Understanding T'ai Chi is to know that it is a health science and not a religion. Yet, T'ai Chi's promotion of quiet mindfulness is beneficial to anyone's spirituality. Therefore, if your church offers T'ai Chi classes, you may enjoy the spiritual focus of the instructor.

Colleges and Universities

Usually T'ai Chi is part of the adult continuing education departments of colleges and universities , although many schools now offer accredited T'ai Chi programs.

In the continuing education departments, these classes are often introductory courses that give you a sample of what T'ai Chi offers. This tendency occurs because colleges require minimum enrollments to continue classes. Since advanced classes are often too small to sustain through colleges, many quality instructors will offer these intro programs so that students can meet them and then continue advanced study through private studio programs.

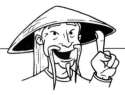

Sage Sifu Says

You should not compare yourself to other students in your T'ai Chi class. Some will be more flexible, some will be less flexible, and none of that matters at all. Lao Tzu said that he who does not contend is beyond reproach. You are always perfect, now and after years of practice.

Support Groups for Health Problems

Many support groups for Parkinson's disease, multiple sclerosis, fibromyalgia, or AIDS (to name a few) may facilitate ongoing T'ai Chi classes for their members. In the Kansas City area, we are working with the local Veterans Hospital to provide T'ai Chi classes specifically geared toward wheelchair practitioners. We are also encouraging hospitals to design rooms with hooks in the ceiling for "climbing harnesses," thereby enabling people with balance disorders to practice T'ai Chi without worrying about falling injuries.

If you are a wheelchair practitioner, you can participate in regular T'ai Chi classes by simply modifying the movements to suit your needs. Interview instructors to find one who can fit your needs. You will need to make your own innovations of the movements if the instructor has no experience with wheelchair students. Also, you may want to take the beginning class more than once since you will have more to cover than your standing peers will.

Everyone with special needs or conditions should contact their local hospitals to request T'ai Chi classes geared to their needs. If you have a support group, organize them to encourage the hospital to innovate. T'ai Chi is about forming lives that fit our needs, and creating your T'ai Chi class can be a great T'ai Chi exercise. Have fun and be creative!

How Do I Choose a Class for Me?

Again, choosing your class depends on your needs. What can you afford? What do you seek to accomplish? Once you decide on the questions to ask, call around and speak to many different instructors. If they are available, take workshops or sample classes through community education programs. This will give you an opportunity to meet the instructors face to face and experience their instruction before enrolling in a long-term class (although most T'ai Chi classes run for only 6 to 10 weeks at a time).

What Is the Cost?

Its helpful to look at T'ai Chi as if it were health insurance. If you pay now with a little money for the class and some time each day to practice, you will reap the benefits for the rest of your life. You will also likely be more productive and make more money in the future. You'll be more relaxed and do less "impulsive" buying, which will save you money, too. T'ai Chi is a very inexpensive investment with a very high return.

The cost of T'ai Chi classes are often determined by the location and by the quality of the instruction. For example, many martial arts studios have longer contracts, which of course requires a larger up-front investment. Each studio is different though, so call and inquire.

No matter what your income level, you will likely be able to find T'ai Chi you can afford. There are many T'ai Chi hobbyists that offer very low cost classes through YMCAs or other community centers. Although these instructors may not be as highly trained as those teaching in the more expensive locations, you can still benefit from attending these classes. Also, higher cost does not guarantee higher-quality instruction. If an instructor has studied for many years, they will likely be better than one who has studied for only a year or two, no matter what the location.

However, to maximize your T'ai Chi experience, you will likely have to pay a bit more. Still, even the highest quality instruction is usually no more than $10 or $15 per class or $80 to $120 per eight-week session (cities vary in cost). In most cities, this is about the cost of a movie, popcorn, and a soda. Not a bad investment for something that can change your life.

T'ai Sci

Research shows that stress costs businesses $7,500 per employee per year, driving up our health care costs. To fight stress–related health costs, some insurance companies and health care providers now pay for or subsidize the cost of T'ai Chi and/or QiGong classes for their clients. Call your insurance carrier to ask if your T'ai Chi class tuition can be rebated or credited on your premiums. Get a receipt from your instructor.

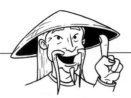

Sage Sifu Says

If you are a member of a senior center or support group, your organization may be eligible for a grant. Available grants may enable you to get very high quality T'ai Chi instruction at little or no cost to participants.

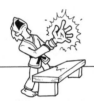

Ouch!

Most people don't practice enough, but don't go berserk and burn yourself out either. Once or twice a day is good for a full session. However, if you're having a tough day at work and want to sneak off for a quick T'ai Chi session in the bathroom or empty boardroom, go for it.

How Often Do I Go?

Different locations will offer different programs, but one T'ai Chi class per week is the most common arrangement. Each class usually runs between an hour to an hour and a half. Some studios may offer two or more classes per week.

There is nothing wrong with going to several classes a week if you can afford it, as long as you don't do it to the point of burn out. However, one class per week is more than enough, as long as you practice at home during the week. In the beginning you may only practice at home for about 10 minutes a day, but over time your practice will get longer as you learn more movements. Eventually you won't have to think about practicing because you'll look forward to it. Whenever you're having a rough day or maybe when you want to celebrate having a good day, you may find yourself slipping out to "play" T'ai Chi. You'll also want to do T'ai Chi when you get home so that you'll be in a better mood to fully enjoy your evening.

Evaluating an Instructor

There are many things to consider as you look for your T'ai Chi instructor. The degrees or awards your potential instructor holds matters very little. More important is whether your instructor's temperament feels good to you. Another consideration is the style of T'ai Chi you want to learn.

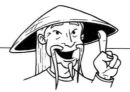

Sage Sifu Says

Because it's new and slow, you may at first find T'ai Chi a little frustrating. This is not uncommon. Remember to breathe and let go of frustrations you feel as you release your breath. Also, you may catch yourself displacing your frustration on the instructor. Be aware that this can happen so don't give up on a good instructor for the wrong reasons. The more you can lighten up on yourself, the more the people around you can lighten up as well, including your instructor.

Instructor Personality

One good question to ask a prospective instructor is, "Do you still study with other T'ai Chi teachers? If a T'ai Chi teacher still studies, it tells you that he/she understands the great depth and endless width of the art and science of T'ai Chi. T'ai Chi expands for a lifetime, just as we expand as living beings, always growing and learning.

Secondly, what is your focus? Are you interested in treating an illness, growing spiritually, or the martial applications of T'ai Chi? The answer to this question will help you know what to ask your prospective instructor. For example, if you have a high-stress corporate career, you may feel comfortable with a T'ai Chi instructor who has experienced that lifestyle and can offer you ways to use the tools he/she teaches in ways meaningful to your life. Or, if your desire is spiritual growth, you may seek an instructor who focuses more on that aspect of T'ai Chi. If you have a particular health problem, you may connect well with a teacher who has the same problem. T'ai Chi is, however, multidimensional in approaches and benefits, so any instructor from any walk of life will be good for you if you feel comfortable and accepted in their presence.

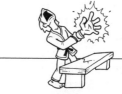

Ouch!

If doing a particular movement doesn't feel right, discuss it with your instructor. Make adjustments on your own as well; everybody does T'ai Chi their own way. Of course there is a proper form, but it takes time for the body to adjust, and for some with injuries or physical conditions that limit movement, although your range of motion will increase, you may never do it just the way your instructor does, and that is perfectly OK. The way you do it is perfect for you.

What I needed personally as a T'ai Chi student was patience. I needed an instructor who didn't scold and patiently allowed me to grow at my own pace. Of course the art of patience is at the core of T'ai Chi, so if your teacher isn't patient on a regular basis, they probably aren't living their T'ai Chi.

You will want a teacher who actually uses the tools they teach and has benefited from them in their lives. You don't want a teacher who's simply teaching because the health club or hospital they work for told them to learn it so they could teach it. If a T'ai Chi teacher is actively using the tools, they are getting better at using them, and they are growing and expanding as a human being, which makes them better at everything they do, including teaching T'ai Chi.

T'ai Chi instruction is not like a regular job. The instructor should be someone who uses the tools and is immersed in the art of personal growth. This doesn't mean that they are some kind of saint. Don't fall into the trap of thinking the T'ai Chi instructor is "above" the trials and tribulations of normal life. A good teacher is someone who lives all that stuff and is lucky enough to have learned the wonderful tools T'ai Chi offers to make the absolute most out of what life offers. A good teacher is therefore not above fear, stress, and worry, but they are learning how to use T'ai Chi to grow as best they can and can communicate to you how they've coped, and how T'ai Chi might help you cope as well.

A T'ai Chi teacher doesn't tell you what's right or how to grow. They explain how the growth tools that T'ai Chi offers has helped them grow. Whatever truth resonates to you is what you take. A T'ai Chi teacher's life, or health, or balance, may not even be as good as yours, but it is much better than it would be if they didn't practice T'ai Chi. Therefore, a T'ai Chi instructor can teach a prize fighter how to punch harder and a basketball star how to shoot better, even though the athlete could soundly defeat the T'ai Chi teacher in their sport. A T'ai Chi teacher teaches the tools of growth, but we all grow in our own ways and at our own pace.

T'ai Chi Styles

The teacher is more important than the style; however, if all teachers are equal, you may decide on a T'ai Chi class by which style you are attracted to. There are several different major T'ai Chi styles. They all have most of the common benefits, and which you choose depends on what looks good to you. The major styles are listed below. Most style names reflect the family name of their original creators.

There are many styles of T'ai Chi and the following list is not comprehensive. It only lists some of the more popular styles. Your local bookstore or the internet are good resources for finding information on a wider selection of T'ai Chi forms.

➤ The extent **Yang Style,** founded by Yang Lu-chan who studied under Chen Style creator Chen Chang-hsing, is widely practiced in the US and China. Yang Lu-chan was eventually invited to teach T'ai Chi to the Imperial Court, and became known as "Yang the Unsurpassed."

➤ The **Kuang Ping Yang Style** of T'ai Chi exhibited in this book, was brought to the United States by Kuo Lien-ying in the 1960's. Kuo trained under Wan Ch'un (a student of Yang Pan-hou, the son of Yang Founder Yang Lu-chan).

➤ The **Chen Style** founder, Chen Chang-hsing, is only four generations removed from T'ai Chi's originator, Cheng San-feng, making the Chen Style closest to the original creator of T'ai Chi. The Chen family split into two forms referred to as the "New Frame" and the "Old Frame." The more extent New Frame is based on the same original 13 postures the Yang, Wu, and Kuang Ping Yang Styles are.

➤ The **Wu Style** was founded by Wu Quan-yu, a student of the originator of the Yang Style, Yang Lu-chan and his son Yang Pan-hou. Wu Quan-yu was Manchurian by race and worked as a bodyguard in the Imperial Court in Beijing. Because of his skill in T'ai Chi and his renown, he did much to help spread knowledge of T'ai Chi Chuan. Some say that the smaller and more restricted movements of the Wu style were due to Master Wu's training in the restrictive clothing of the Imperial Court, and would therefore be an ideal self-defense training for use in modern street clothes.

➤ **Mulan Quan** is a modern form, founded by Sifu Mei Fing Ying. Mulan is named after the legendary young woman Fa Mulan (who's name translates to "wooden orchid"). Besides its basic hand form, Mulan Quan offers a Sword Style as do some other forms and also a somewhat unique Fan Style. Although derived from the nearly extinct form, Hua Chia Chan, its founder simplified its forms and added more *wushu* (martial arts). The form was approved by martial arts masters and named Mulan Quan in 1988.

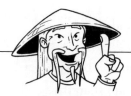

Sage Sifu Says

Every style can be done by everybody. If 30 different people are in a room doing the same style, you'll see 30 different ways to do it because we all move differently. A good instructor will realize this and may correct a way you are doing it, but will accept it when you say, "My body doesn't do it that way, yet, but I'm working on it." So, while always striving for perfection being continually contented with where you are, grounded in the reality *that you are always evolving perfect.*

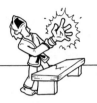

Ouch!

If you have arthritis or a balance disorder, be cautious of the "fast" forms. It doesn't mean they are bad for you, but you have to be your own best advisor as to what you want to do. Listen to your body; do what feels right.

Each style varies a bit depending on the instructor. T'ai Chi is a living art, and it changes and grows as it is passed down through the generations. The Chinese masters said, "learn T'ai Chi exactly as you are taught, your personality will polish it effortlessly." So, for example, even if you study Yang style T'ai Chi, your forms will likely be a bit different from other schools of the same style. No one is wrong or right, just different. Just as each rose has its own *unique* beauty, but each is beautiful. It would be comical for a rose to strut around the garden proclaiming that its beauty was superior.

However, there are certain tenets that all T'ai Chi adheres to and must be observed by all students. Some concepts include the dan tien, vertical axis, effortless flexibility, and mindfulness, which will be discussed in detail later in Chapter 9.

Some styles have modified "fast" versions. In fact, all T'ai Chi can be done at varying speeds, and it is fun to experiment with different rhythms and speeds. However, in class your instructor will probably move quite slowly. Some styles also offer advanced students variations that use swords or fans.

The Least You Need to Know

➤ T'ai Chi classes can be found almost anywhere.

➤ No matter your needs, a class can be found to fill them.

➤ No matter what your budget is, T'ai Chi is affordable.

➤ Ask your insurance carrier if they pay for T'ai Chi.

➤ Attend class weekly and practice daily.

➤ The best instructor for you is one you like.

➤ The best style is the one that looks fun to you.

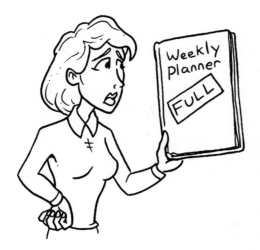

Where and When?

Chapter 7 will explain where and when to do T'ai Chi, as well as what to wear. You will discover that these questions are not only a matter of etiquette or convenience, but can also affect the health benefits you get from T'ai Chi.

You will discover the advantages of a large class vs. private instruction, video/book instruction vs. live classes, and also tips on how to make time for whatever T'ai Chi program you choose.

Do It Yourself at Home

Although practicing at home by yourself on a regular basis is how T'ai Chi's benefits are realized, studying with a qualified instructor is an essential part of the success of your home practice. No matter how many years you study T'ai Chi, you can still benefit from studying in classes. T'ai Chi, like life, is an endless growth process.

Most of us in the modern world want fast answers. We like to take classes or workshops and move on. And sometimes our educational motivation has more to do with getting our hands on a piece of paper that says we know something, than with personally being changed by the knowledge.

Therefore, most people rush through a T'ai Chi course to learn a few moves and then think they are done. Of course, you do get some benefit from any exposure to T'ai Chi. You can learn things on the first day that can benefit the rest of your life. But, why stop there? T'ai Chi can offer you a deep ocean of experience. After 20 years of T'ai Chi practice, I still study with my instructor, and even though the very first class was beneficial and wonderful, I still find benefit that carries into my home practice in each and every class.

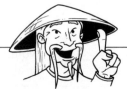

Sage Sifu Says

If you get frustrated by a class and drop out, don't make it a life sentence. Keep coming back to T'ai Chi. Each class will make you more confident. Repeat the beginner class as many times as you like; there are no deadlines or expectations in T'ai Chi. Relax. Take your time. Play.

T'ai Chi provides life-long benefits and should be practiced for the rest of our lives. However, this isn't a marriage contract. Don't feel smothered by this. Drop in and out of T'ai Chi as often as you like. T'ai Chi will always be patiently waiting for you when you come back, like a touchstone or a port in a storm. Eventually you will do T'ai Chi simply because you feel pretty spectacular when you do. Besides finding classes personally enjoyable, you will discover that T'ai Chi attracts interesting people, and the social aspect will draw you as well.

Bookworm T'ai Chi

T'ai Chi books are great for helping you understand the philosophy, art, and science of T'ai Chi, and as supplements to classes. However, a book cannot replace a live instructor or the other benefits of a class.

It is difficult in books to explain how the body moves through movements because books are dependent on still photographs. The ability to see an instructor move and to ask for clarification or hear the questions of other students is invaluable. Also, it is easier in person for instructors to explain things in stages while you relax, whereas when using a book, facts must be remembered because the instructor isn't there to remind you.

Video T'ai Chi

If you do not have access to T'ai Chi classes, a video is the next best way to learn. Also, you can use books to supplement your understanding of what videos teach. Using books and videos together can help maximize the benefit of your T'ai Chi practice. As the videos teach visually and audibly enabling your mind to relax, the books round out your intellectual understanding of the movements and exercises.

Consider that the average 8-week introductory T'ai Chi class entails at least 12 hours of instruction. The average T'ai Chi video is 1 hour. You can see that it is difficult for an instructor to explain a 2,000-year-old art and science that is so rich in benefits in a 1-hour video. Some videos are done in multivolume, several-hour sets, which is the best way to go if you do not have access to live T'ai Chi classes. Your author, Bill Douglas, offers multivolume T'ai Chi video courses for individuals and corporate wellness programs in the back of this book. These are great if you have no access to live classes, but again go for the live class if you can.

Videos can be great supplements to your ongoing T'ai Chi class, especially if your instructor has produced one or approves one for the class. Be aware however that even if a video covers the same style you are studying, the style may look different. If you are in a class, check with your instructor before purchasing a video. Bookstores, magazine ads, and martial arts stores are usually good places to find an assortment of T'ai Chi videos.

Outdoor vs. Indoor

The single most important thing about practicing T'ai Chi is that you actually do practice it. Where you practice is secondary. The following recommendation to do T'ai Chi outdoors should not be construed to mean that you should not practice inside. If you can do T'ai Chi outdoors, do so. However, if you don't feel comfortable doing it outside because of where you live or the weather, then by all means do it inside.

Outdoor T'ai Chi

The purpose of T'ai Chi and other QiGong exercises is to promote the flow of Qi. Qi's life energy flows through us and all living things. Therefore, the Chinese have always advocated performing T'ai Chi outdoors where you can enjoy and benefit from the Qi of other living things. In fact, Traditional Chinese Medicine teaches that when we do T'ai Chi, our relaxed body and mind benefit from nature's healing energy even more.

We all know that just being in nature has a soothing quality, so if T'ai Chi can magnify this benefit, all the better. The word "mesmerize" is derived from the name of the famous Dr. Mesma. Dr. Mesma worked with patients suffering from psychotic episodes. Reportedly, Dr. Mesma would instruct his patients to sit with their backs up against a tree whenever they felt an episode coming on, and his patients were said to benefit greatly from this "nature therapy."

As you practice T'ai Chi in your backyard, the park, or even around the plants in your house, you may experience the benefits of this therapy for yourself.

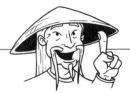

Sage Sifu Says

Your balance fluctuates from day to day, yet like a bullish stock market it is always improving. So, on days when your balance is at its worst, don't think you are not benefiting from T'ai Chi. Rather, let go of constantly measuring your progress. Enjoy your loss of balance even as much as you enjoy the T'ai Chi on days when your balance is great.

Surfaces

T'ai Chi should be practiced on a level, predictable surface, especially when you are beginning. As you play over the years, you may experiment with more uneven and challenging surfaces.

T'ai Chi can be performed on grass, sand, dirt, or pavement. It is good to practice on varying types of surfaces because this gives your mind/body communication even more information for improving your balance.

Try to choose a flat area, out of direct sunlight. Soft morning sunlight or evening light is all right, but do not practice in direct sunlight during the hot part of the day. You will discover that practicing T'ai Chi in different light is challenging as well. Doing T'ai Chi in the dimming light of sunset challenges you to use more internal and less external balance references.

Indoor T'ai Chi

The benefits of doing T'ai Chi indoors are pretty obvious if it's freezing, smoldering hot, or the mosquito population is in full production. Though outdoors is optimum, T'ai Chi benefits can be had anywhere and anytime.

Again, when we are having a tough day at the office, it's great to slip off to the restroom or the supply room to drift into a T'ai Chi getaway. If you practice T'ai Chi at home before work or in the evening, it is often just more convenient to practice inside.

One problem students encounter indoors is space. As you move through your T'ai Chi repertoire, you often will cover more ground than your living room provides. If the next step takes you through a wall, just remember where you are at, move back a couple steps, and pick up where you left off. Eventually, you won't even think about it. T'ai Chi pours into your living room, just like it easily and naturally flows into your life. Just as T'ai Chi encourages an almost liquid relaxation of mind and body, its use and benefits can seem to pour into every nook and cranny of our lives with much benefit.

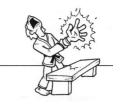

Ouch!

When you run out of room doing T'ai Chi, you adjust by moving back two steps and resuming. Most people live in cities, and this "apartment T'ai Chi" is how most T'ai Chi must be done. Don't psych yourself into thinking you cannot practice T'ai Chi because your house isn't big enough. These are not limitations but opportunities to learn flexibility in mind as well as body.

The Horary Clock

Acupuncture, Chinese herbal medicine, and T'ai Chi understand that the body has natural rhythms that align with certain organs and functions. You can actually use this "horary" (hourly) clock to treat problems. Each organ has certain hours called peak hours. These peak hours are generally the best for treating these organs and are listed in the chart below:

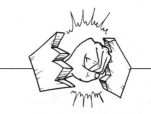

A T'ai Chi Punch Line

When doing T'ai Chi indoors, you should minimize noise by turning off the TV and stereo; don't let noises beyond your control be an issue. Noise is in the ear of the beholder.

➤ 11 A.M. to 1 P.M. Heart

➤ 1 P.M. to 3 P.M. Small Intestine

➤ 3 P.M. to 5 P.M. Bladder

➤ 5 P.M. to 7 P. M. Kidney

➤ 7 P.M. to 9 P.M. Pericardium

➤ 9 P.M. to 11 P.M. Triple Burner

➤ 11 P.M. to 1 A.M. Gallbladder

➤ 1 A.M. to 3 A.M. Liver

➤ 3 A.M. to 5 A.M. Lung

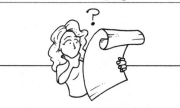

➤ 5 A.M. to 7 A.M. Large Intestine

➤ 7 A.M. to 9 A.M. Stomach

➤ 9 A.M. to 11 A.M. Spleen

In Part 3, I will introduce some QiGong exercises for specific organs. However, T'ai Chi can generally tonify all the aspects of the body and every organ. Therefore, T'ai Chi practice at a peak hour could provide a good therapy. Yet, if your peak hour is in the middle of the night, you may prefer a sitting or lying QiGong exercise to focus Qi into the desired organ. The sitting QiGong exercise in Part 3 will give you a great technique to use in peak hours.

Large Class vs. Private Class

Surprisingly, learning in a large class has several advantages over more expensive private lessons, although both have their own strengths, depending on your needs.

Private Lesson's Pros and Cons

Very few people get private lessons. Part of the reason is that they can be very expensive. A good T'ai Chi instructor usually will begin at about $75 per hour and can go up significantly from there.

However some people, such as emergency room physicians, have erratic, demanding schedules and are forced to take private lessons. This is a highly effective way to learn the T'ai Chi forms in a very short period of time because the instructor's entire focus is on your learning.

Private lessons can also be beneficial to those learning to be instructors, thereby enabling them to learn minute details and background on movements and their purpose.

Know Your Chinese

In Traditional Chinese Medicine, the word **tonify** means to strengthen, to energize, and to imbue with health. Therefore, it can be applied to Qi, blood, tissue, organs, or processes in the body or mind.

T'ai Sci

Any malady should be discussed with a physician. However, in addition to your medical doctor, you may want to discuss your condition with a certified doctor of Traditional Chinese Medicine. Using QiGong on your own can be a powerful adjunct therapy for a condition you may be treating; however if used under the direction of a Traditional Chinese Medical practitioner, it may be even more effectively used.

Large Classes

If an instructor is in great demand, their classes will inevitably be larger. Therefore, you will get less personal attention but will benefit from their quality of instruction. On the other hand you may find instructors in less demand with smaller classes that can provide you with more personal instruction. Decide what your priorities are and then choose a class size that meets your needs.

You can learn very effectively in a large class setting. In fact, there are distinct advantages to being in a large class. As fellow classmates ask questions for clarification, you can benefit by their inquiries. Also, you will discover that there is a group energy to T'ai Chi classes. Just as plants emit life energy, so do other people, and as your classmates practice T'ai Chi, you can bask in the glow of their presence.

Usually, an accomplished T'ai Chi instructor will have numerous advanced students who will help as assistants. In a larger class, you can benefit from the expertise these students have to offer. Note that advanced students probably are less than perfect, but so is the instructor. You will learn T'ai Chi in layers, and the advanced students can give you a layer of instruction that the instructor can add to or polish over the months and years.

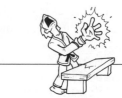

Ouch!

Do not assume the instructor is aware of a problem you have with a movement or the class program. Ask questions during class to clarify instruction. However, if you have concerns about the program, discuss it with the instructor after class. Before you stop attending a T'ai Chi class in frustration, discuss concerns with the instructor. Most instructors want to help you get it—that's why they're there.

T'ai Chi classes will benefit you even if you take them for a short time, providing you with tools you can use for the rest of your life. However, it is best to take classes for a lifetime. It is fun, beneficial, and a great way to meet interesting people, so why not? By doing so, you have no deadline or rush to progress at a certain speed. If you practice everyday for a few minutes you will likely learn the forms quite easily. However, if you need to repeat the beginning class again, and again, that is no problem.

If you are in a large class, you may have to move around a bit to see what the instructor is doing. Move to wherever you need to be to see. T'ai Chi is very informal. Usually, in a very large class there will be advanced students positioned in various locations so that you can follow them if you cannot see the instructor clearly. If you aren't sure what is being taught, raise your hand and ask for clarification. Don't be shy about this. The best T'ai Chi classes are ones where students interact and ask questions. The least productive classes are those where the teacher does all the talking.

Making Time for QiGong and T'ai Chi Class and Practice

To maximize your benefit of T'ai Chi practice, it's best to spend about 20 minutes in the morning doing T'ai Chi or a sitting QiGong meditation exercise. Spend another

20 minutes in the evening doing whichever one you didn't do in the morning. Usually the first response to this suggestion is, "I don't have an extra 40 minutes a day!"

If that is your response, ask yourself the following questions:

➤ Do you spend 40 minutes a day watching television?

➤ Do you spend your morning and afternoon breaks drinking soda or coffee and chatting?

➤ Do you ever spend time anxiously waiting to access the internet, or waiting for the computer to print, or dinner to bake?

For most of us, the answer to at least one of these questions is yes. This shows you that you probably do have an extra 40 minutes a day. So, the main difficulty in doing T'ai Chi isn't really having the time, but deciding to do it. When we decide to do it, we find that we make time. Beginning new life habits is one of the single most difficult things people attempt. But T'ai Chi is worth it.

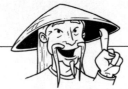

Sage Sifu Says

Because T'ai Chi practice calms us and clears our mind, it actually creates extra time. When we are calmer and clearer we are more efficient, we are easier to live with, and we find it easier to relax and sleep. So the 40 or 50 minutes we spend on T'ai Chi and QiGong can save us hours in effort and frustration.

Life Habits Are Hard to Change

T'ai Chi is new for you. You will find that it will take time to get used to doing it every day. Don't punish or scold yourself when you forget. Just enjoy it when you do do it. The following example will help you see just how difficult it is to change life habits, so you can go easy on yourself as you begin to adapt to a new life with T'ai Chi.

A study of cardiac recovery patients shows just how difficult it is to change. Patients were given a choice of two therapies to follow after their heart attacks. The first was only to take medication and be released within days. Unfortunately, that first choice carried a prognosis of another possible major heart attack within a few months. The second choice involved staying in the hospital for a much longer period to learn stress management techniques and new dietary changes and offered a much rosier forecast of the patients likely going several years before another coronary. Amazingly, nearly all the patients opted to leave immediately, even though it increased the likelihood of a premature death.

What is ironic about T'ai Chi is that even though it may be difficult to incorporate into your life at first, it will make all other healthy life changes much easier. Again, T'ai Chi is a technology designed to help us change with less effort and stress. Therefore, the longer we practice T'ai Chi, the easier it is for us to change. So, if you decide to go on a healthier diet, stop smoking, or start getting out in nature more, the effort you make to learn T'ai Chi will make all these other efforts to change more "effortless."

T'ai Chi Is Positively Effortless

Studies show that when we change for positive reasons, we are much more likely to change our habits. Therefore, rather than do T'ai Chi because your blood pressure is high or your stress levels are unbearable, do T'ai Chi because it feels good. Don't rush through your T'ai Chi, but make it a little oasis in your busy day. Slow down enough to feel the pleasure of the movement and the stretches. Enjoy how good it feels to breathe deeply and let the whole body relax. This will condition you day by day to love the feeling T'ai Chi gives you, causing you to look forward to it and miss it when you don't do it.

Make a Calendar

Create a T'ai Chi calendar and place it on your refrigerator door. Every time you do your T'ai Chi or QiGong, mark a big X on that day's square. As you begin to get a few days in a row, you will want to keep that string going. You will also begin to notice that the more Xs you have on the calendar, the better you feel. Your awareness becomes more subtle and pleasant, which will help you make the transition from doing T'ai Chi for the calendar accomplishment to doing it for how it makes you feel.

Ouch!

When you forget to do T'ai Chi, don't scold yourself. Our mind plays funny games to keep from growing and changing. Making ourselves "bad" for not immediately adopting new life habits is one of those games. If you forgot to do T'ai Chi, just relax and do it now—no big deal. Breathe and enjoy.

Social T'ai Chi

T'ai Chi clubs are increasingly popular in the United States, as they have been in China for centuries. This is because even though T'ai Chi is a terrific personal exercise and is thoroughly enjoyable alone, it can also be a terrific social event. There is a group energy that T'ai Chi clubs offer that can heighten the pleasure T'ai Chi provides.

T'ai Chi clubs also are very supportive and encourage T'ai Chi players to practice on their own. When we have a class or a club to get together with, we are much more likely to practice on our own at home. We want to improve our T'ai Chi so that we can play more complex T'ai Chi games using mirror image forms and other games involving several players. Therefore, continuing with a T'ai Chi class or club for the rest of your life is a great way to stick with T'ai Chi for the long haul. Social T'ai Chi is also terrific since T'ai Chi practice can extend your life substantially; if you outlive all your peers you won't be lonely because you'll still have your T'ai Chi club to hang out with.

The Least You Need to Know

➤ If you don't have access to live classes, videos and books can be used.

➤ Although outdoor T'ai Chi is optimum, indoor T'ai Chi is great, too.

➤ Treat certain organs by using the "Horary" Clock.

➤ Large classes can be great if you ask questions.

➤ Use a calendar to get used to practicing, until T'ai Chi becomes an integral part of your life.

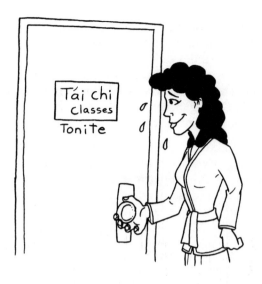

The First Day of Class

In This Chapter

➤ What to wear to class

➤ Preparing mentally & physically for class

➤ How T'ai Chi is taught

➤ What is expected of you?

➤ Learn the terms

Here you will learn what to wear to do T'ai Chi. Yet, beyond fashion concerns, Chapter 8 will also prepare you mentally, emotionally, and physically for your first day of class. Even those currently involved in T'ai Chi will find these mental and emotional insights into T'ai Chi challenges helpful.

This chapter will provide you with many ways to get the most out of T'ai Chi training by explaining class structure, what is expected of you, and clarifying terms you may encounter in class.

The T'ai Chi Wardrobe

Here you will learn what to wear to T'ai Chi class. (Ultimately you can do T'ai Chi in any kind of clothing, but certain clothing *is* suggested for class.) Usually, T'ai Chi students wear anything they want. It is helpful to wear something loose and stretchy

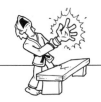

and to leave jewelry at home; however, the rest is often up to you. The most common T'ai Chi suit is a T-shirt and sweat pants. Spandex or body suits, although not prohibited, are not typically worn in T'ai Chi. Also, longer dresses can make it more difficult for an instructor to see posture or leg placement, but if your class is in an office environment at work, don't worry about it.

If you practice T'ai Chi at the office, everyone will likely be wearing office clothes, but they will kick off their heels. If you go from the office to a studio or community class or if your company holds classes in an exercise area, bring some sweats and tennis shoes to change into.

Some studios, especially martial arts studios may require more formal attire. If they do, they will direct you to a martial arts supply store that sells them, or the studio may provide them.

Footwear depends on the location. For most T'ai Chi classes, tennis shoes are fine. However, some studios that offer T'ai Chi, such as martial arts or yoga studios, will require bare feet. It is not advisable to wear only socks in these studios because socks can be slippery. If you need arch support and attend a class in these locations, you may be able to wear tennis shoes that have never been used on the street or Chinese kung fu shoes. These nonstreet shoes will not damage the floor, but check with the instructor before purchasing them.

The only hard and fast rule that all instructors follow on footwear is that you cannot wear heeled shoes. This is hard on your back, makes balance difficult, and changes the way the whole body moves. If doing T'ai Chi at the office, just kick off your heels or bring tennis shoes for T'ai Chi if that feels more comfortable.

External and Internal Hygiene

T'ai Chi has very few external hygiene rules, but internally, it is good to prepare yourself mentally and emotionally by letting go of some myths about yourself and exercise.

External Hygiene

Unlike most other martial arts, T'ai Chi usually requires no contact between participants. Therefore, hygiene rules are pretty much like daily life. You will be in fairly close proximity to others, so if your job leaves you a little ripe, you may want to shower prior to T'ai Chi class. However, if you come to class from the office, there shouldn't be a problem. The only concern might be if you attend class at a studio that requires you to go barefoot. If you go straight from the office to one of these classes, you might just buy some handy-wipe wet towelettes and clean your feet off prior to going into class.

Don't wear heavy cologne or perfume into class because the deep breathing in T'ai Chi may make it overwhelming to others. Again, jewelry should be left at home, especially jangley jewelry.

Internal Hygiene

The clutter in our minds, hearts, and body is the most important thing to cleanse prior to attending your first—or one hundredth—T'ai Chi class.

In the long run T'ai Chi will help relieve allergy problems, but if you have heavy allergies and are heavily medicated, it may be helpful to lighten up on the medications prior to T'ai Chi. That is, if your medications make your balance more difficult or make it harder to focus. However, never adjust prescription medication without your doctor's approval. If you haven't tried acupuncture for your allergies, try it. It can be a terrific nonpharmaceutical way to alleviate allergy symptoms with great results. Acupuncture treatments cannot harm, but can enhance your clarity or balance.

T'ai Chi & Massage Therapy

T'ai Chi is meant to loosen the mind and body and increase internal awareness. Tension disconnects the mind from the body. Therefore, you may find it very complimentary to begin massage therapy prior to your first T'ai Chi class and to continue massage therapy for the rest of your life. Most good T'ai Chi teachers will advocate massage therapy as part of your T'ai Chi training, just as many good massage therapists will recommend T'ai Chi to their clients. You also will find that massage therapy will be helpful in relieving chronic problems such as allergies.

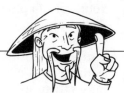

Sage Sifu Says

As T'ai Chi teaches the body to move and change more easily and effortlessly, it provides a model for the mind and heart to change more easily, too. Therefore, as you continue with T'ai Chi, you may discover you eat healthier, drink more water and less soda, get better rest, adopt habits like regular massage therapy, and spend more time with people who make you feel good about yourself.

Resistance to Change

T'ai Chi helps us change. Our mind and body get accustomed to the way we have always done things, even things that are not really that good for us. Therefore, on a subconscious level, parts of us resist good changes that T'ai Chi fosters because we don't want to let go of the way we have always been. Part of us likes to be a "couch potato" and doesn't like the way T'ai Chi is getting us more involved in an active life. Resistance to change may manifest itself in many ways.

Resistance may do the following:

➤ Cause you to scold yourself, to tell yourself you are too clumsy, too uncoordinated, too slow, or too tired to do T'ai Chi.

➤ Tell you T'ai Chi is for *other people* who are better, smarter, stronger, or more coordinated than you are.

➤ Tell you that the teacher doesn't like you or that T'ai Chi is dumb and useless.

➤ Tell you that it would be much more fun to watch TV and eat potato chips tonight, *rather than going all the way out to your T'ai Chi class.*

➤ If you miss a class, resistance will tell you, "You're already too far behind; *don't go back there.*"

If you hang in there long enough, however, you will discover that after nearly every T'ai Chi class, you will feel much better than you did before going. If you become conscious of the voices of "resistance," you will be more likely to stick with T'ai Chi.

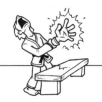

Ouch!

Students often obsess on remembering each detail the instructor tells them; some even bring a pad and pencil to class. Don't do that. Relax. Good instructors will repeat important things over and over. Let yourself enjoy the class. Don't make T'ai Chi class another "important," "serious" thing in your life. Let it be playtime.

"Wrongness" Is Our Culture's "Resistance"

Your T'ai Chi progress will be held back by something that affects our entire culture. If you understand this, it will take a great deal of pressure off of you and your instructor. Most Western students are obsessed with learning the T'ai Chi movements "perfectly," and this causes them stress, which slows their ability to learn and enjoy T'ai Chi. In fact, we often convince ourselves that our attempts to learn are so "imperfect" that it is pointless to continue with our study.

T'ai Chi will show you on a very basic level that you are never "wrong." You are growing and learning how to do things better and better each and every day of your life. T'ai Chi is simple enough to use the very first day of practice, but its richness is so subtle that you can refine your T'ai Chi movements for the rest of your life.

Therefore, you do not need to "perfect" the first movement before learning the second. You learn a layer of the movements, and learning that layer changes who you are and how you function. Your new and improved self can then learn the movements at yet a deeper, more subtle level, and so on for years and years. T'ai Chi leaves you in an endlessly blooming state of perfection.

Your First Class

When entering your first class, you probably aren't sure what it will look like, how to treat the instructor, or what is expected of you. So, let's look at these expectations one at a time.

Mainly, you will be expected to relax and enjoy yourself. You will also have a little homework, but as you'll see, this could be the best homework you ever had.

Addressing Your Instructor

The question of how to address your instructor has several possible answers. The safest way to find out what is right for the class you enroll in is to simply ask the teacher how they would like to be addressed. The formal Chinese term for T'ai Chi teacher is *Sifu* (pronounced *see-foo*), meaning master of an art or skill. However, many T'ai Chi classes in the West are very informal. Most instructors simply go by their first name.

If a Chinese teacher asks you to call him or her Sifu, this is not because of an ego trip. Actually, this is a great compliment. This means that they consider you a worthy student, and that is an honor. They are paying you a compliment by asking you to call them Sifu.

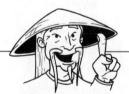

Sage Sifu Says

You can get all the benefits from T'ai Chi without straining. You don't have to memorize all the terms, or do the movements exactly like your teacher does, or read any certain books. T'ai Chi's amazing benefits will come to you by simply breathing deeply, relaxing your mind, and playing T'ai Chi in class and every day at home. Play T'ai Chi every day, and everything else will take care of itself.

Class Structure

T'ai Chi is informal, and each class is different. Some classes begin with a sitting QiGong exercise, using chairs forming a circle. For this relaxation exercise, the instructor will likely lead the group through an imagery exercise as they sit quietly with their eyes closed. Other classes will not use chairs and may begin with a standing relaxation exercise, also with the students' eyes closed. Still other instructors may begin the class by leading students in warm up exercises without practicing a QiGong or relaxation exercise.

Ouch!

Your main goal in T'ai Chi class should be to relax and breathe. By not trying too hard, you learn more easily. Students who frustrate themselves by mentally repeating that they "can't get it" usually prove themselves right. If you really can't learn the movement, just follow the other students as you breathe and relax. You'll feel good after class, and you can repeat the session again, and you'll be the expert in class the second time around.

Once relaxation exercises are done, the physical class structure will probably have students staggered throughout the room facing the instructor in lines. The instructor usually faces the class, which forms lines throughout the room, giving each student enough space to swing their arms without striking one another. However, smaller, more informal classes may form a circle. An instructor may alternate facing the class or with his/her back to the class, and may move around the room as well giving students different angles to see from.

In a class formed in lines facing the instructor, find a place where you can see what the instructor is doing. Many large classes will have advanced students to help, and you can watch them if you can't see the instructor. If you can't see what's going on, ask questions or change places. Be clear of your needs. The teachers want to help you understand the movements, but in a larger class, they may not know you need further explanation. Be assertive—they want to help you understand.

The list below gives you an idea of the process a T'ai Chi class might go through, however each instructor has their own format.

➤ Sitting or Standing Relaxation Exercise (if your class performs these).

➤ T'ai Chi warm up exercises—gentle, repetitive movements that prepare you physically and mentally for T'ai Chi (many warm ups are moving QiGong exercises and are discussed in detail in Part 3).

➤ After warm ups, the instructor may teach individual movements to practice or if he/she teaches by exhibition, they will begin performing the entire T'ai Chi set and you will be expected to follow along.

➤ Your homework is the movements themselves, although it is highly recommended to begin using the QiGong relaxation exercises at home for your own health and pleasure.

T'ai Chi usually does not require anyone to sit or lie on the floor; however, some instructors may have warm up or cool down exercises that require it. If you are unable to do so because of an injury or physical limitation, discuss alternatives with the instructor.

How Are T'ai Chi Movements Taught?

T'ai Chi forms involve a series of choreographed martial arts poses that flow together like a slow motion dance. How these movements are taught can vary. Some classes are taught by example. Meaning, the instructor will lead the group all the way through the entire T'ai Chi form, and the students mimic until over time they remember all the movements.

However, many classes are taught for different levels, whereby the movements are broken down into one or two movements per class. If you are an average learner, these classes are preferable. It is much easier to learn one movement at a time and practice it all week than it is to try to assimilate an entire T'ai Chi form. I'll mention here that your learning will be much easier if you don't miss classes. It's easier to memorize movements in smaller bites. For each class you miss the bites get larger.

The points below lay out how T'ai Chi is taught or might be studied, in an effort to help you get the most out of your classes.

➤ Warm ups and relaxation techniques are usually repeated weekly, although if you practice these everyday on your own you will be all the better for it.

➤ The actual T'ai Chi movement of the week must be learned and practiced on your own that week.

➤ Each week a new T'ai Chi movement will be added to your growing form or repertoire.

➤ The form will get longer and longer each week until you learn the entire form.

➤ Long forms of 20 minutes take between 6 and 8 months to learn.

➤ Short forms of 10 minutes may take 2 to 6 months to learn, depending on the instructor and the form.

➤ Advanced students often repeat beginning or intermediate classes for years to refine their performance of the T'ai Chi forms.

➤ Advanced students may serve as assistant instructors in class.

➤ As an advanced student you may be asked to assist new students learning the forms for the first time. T'ai Chi like all martial arts is based on a mentoring system.

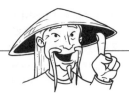

Sage Sifu Says

Normal T'ai Chi exercises can be easily adjusted to conform to your living room's size. However, the more advanced sword or fan forms that some styles teach, although more challenging, can easily be done indoors, too. For example, retractable swords are available and can be left retracted when practicing indoors.

The bottom line is, you can always practice T'ai Chi, no matter what style or where you are.

You Mean There's Homework!?!

T'ai Chi class exposes you to the movements, then you must practice those movements at home. There are two ways to look at this: either as another burden on your life's full plate, or as a chance to take a break from the rat race and let all the weight of the world roll right off your shoulders.

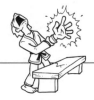

Ouch!

At first it will be difficult to discipline yourself to practice daily. If you fall behind in class, just play along and repeat the multiweek session again. There are no deadlines. You'll get it eventually. Don't sabotage yourself into thinking you just can't get it. Regular attendance and daily practice makes T'ai Chi effortless and fruitful. If you miss class, although some instructors may help you catch up individually, you can't expect it.

The very first movement you learn on the very first day of class is a fantastic QiGong relaxation exercise that can help you begin to dump stress, if you do it in the right frame of mind. If you only do the T'ai Chi movement to prepare for the next T'ai Chi class, it won't be that relaxing. However, if you breathe deeply and let every muscle of your body relax, allowing the burdens of the week to roll off your shoulders each time you practice the movement, it'll feel great!

To learn T'ai Chi, you will need to practice at home. But, the reason we learn T'ai Chi is because it feels good, so why wouldn't we want to practice something that makes us feel good.

T'ai Chi Etiquette

Most instructors are happy to get questions during class. The rest of the class, or at least some of them, are probably facing the same uncertainties or challenges as you. A good instructor has been studying many years and may not remember all the challenges new students have, so your inquiries help him to help you and the other students. If your questions are criticisms of the format or structure, it would be best to offer them to the instructor personally after class. The instructor may not be able to fix it, but he may explain why it is done the way it is.

Martial Terms for T'ai Chi

Since T'ai Chi was originally a martial art, an introduction to some martial arts terms may be helpful. When you learn T'ai Chi, your instructor may use these or similar terms to describe the T'ai Chi movements. Understand that any one of these martial arts movements can be done any way that you need to do it for your own comfort. So, if you have an injury or condition that limits your movement, do it in a way that feels comfortable to you. Never strain yourself to do something that doesn't feel right; just modify it a bit, kick lower, or reach less. As you play T'ai Chi in a way that feels good, over the days, months, and years, your kicks will get higher and higher.

Punches

In T'ai Chi there are punches. They are not hard grunting punches, but soft relaxing punches. There are generally three types of punches used. Both punches illustrated in the following figures begin with your fist by your hip, with the palm side of the fist turned up toward the sky. The first, is a common T'ai Chi punch and begins with the fist at waist, palm turned in toward body, with no rotation of the fist as you punch. The other two are slightly more complex and therefore shown in the following figures. However, one then does a full twist as you send it out to punch in front of you, so the fist ends up with the palm facing down to the ground.

The second punch is a Half Twist Punch. This begins with the fist near the hip with the palm turned up. When you throw the punch

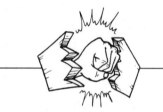

A T'ai Chi Punch Line

Many of the movements in T'ai Chi have martial arts applications, and were patterned after the movements of creatures or images in nature. Therefore, T'ai Chi movements serve practical self-defense purposes and simultaneously are soothing natural motions which encourage the flow of Qi through the body just as Qi flows through all of nature.

out, the fist rotates only a half turn, leaving the knuckles lined up in a row, top knuckle toward the sky and pinkie knuckle toward the ground.

In the Full Fist Turn Punch, the fist ends up palm down.

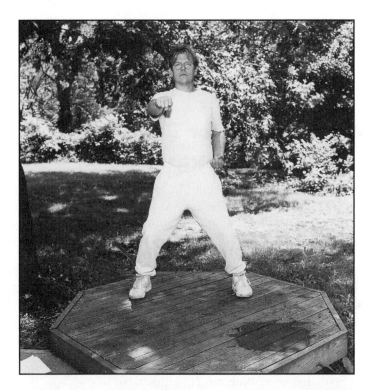

The Half Twist Punch is more common in T'ai Chi, with knuckles ending up vertical.

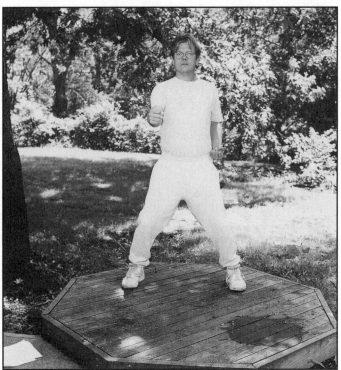

Punches are generally not thrown out in big circular haymaker punches like John Wayne threw. They come straight out from the hip like a piston, with the elbows tucked in. The elbows usually don't extend out from the sides, but stay in near the body.

Because of the many Western movies we've seen, most Westerners also try to punch with the whole upper body, actually leaning into the punch. However, in T'ai Chi and all martial arts, you do not normally lean into the punch. When the punch is complete, your head will still be posturally aligned above the dan tien.

Although there may be exceptions to how punches are thrown in various T'ai Chi forms, usually the rule of not leaning forward is always observed. However, there are times when the fist may circle around, rather than punch straight out from the hip. In Part Four, you will see an example of this in the "Box Opponent's Ears" movement.

The Ins and Outs of Blocking

There are three types of blocks, In Blocks, Out Blocks, and Up Blocks. Their names explain whether the arm is blocking in toward the center of your body, out away from the center of your body, or up away from the body. One other less-used block is the Down Block, which looks like an Out Block in reverse. An example is seen in Part 4's "Wind Blowing Lotus Leaves" movement.

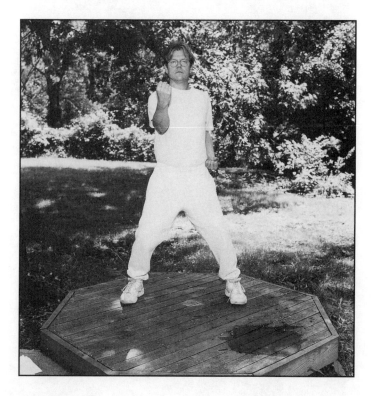

An In Block begins with the fist near your ear and then pull the arm in a circular motion across the front of your body.

An Out Block begins with the fist near your groin, and then pull the arm in a circular sweep up across the body to block outward.

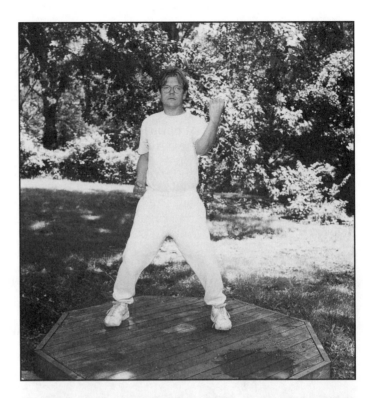

An Up Block begins with the fist palm facing your face, and then twist the palm away up to the sky, blocking up and away.

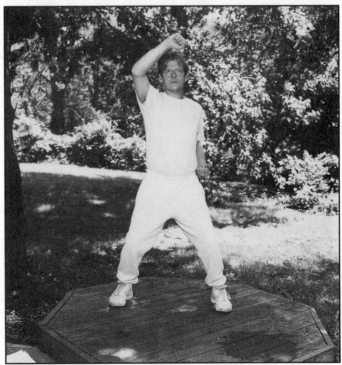

Getting Your Kicks

T'ai Chi generally uses three kicks, Side or Separation Kicks, Crescent Kicks, or Front Kicks. Examples of these kicks can be viewed in Part 4, where the side kick is called "Separation of the Right Foot (and left foot)," the Crescent Kick is called "Wave Hand Over Water Lily Kick," and the Front Kick is called "Front Kick."

The Least You Need to Know

➤ Ask the class instructor what to wear.

➤ T'ai Chi can encourage healthful lifestyle changes, such as massages or nondrug treatments for health problems.

➤ T'ai Chi makes life changes easier.

➤ Instructors will tell you what is expected of you.

➤ Practice because it feels good.

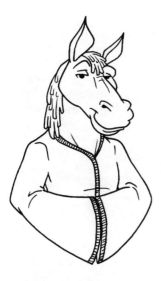

Horse Stance and Other Terms— Saddle Up!

In This Chapter

➤ Understand the importance of T'ai Chi posture

➤ How T'ai Chi protects your joints

➤ T'ai Chi's moves teach effortless living

➤ Breath is the beginning of everything

Chapter 9 explains the core concepts that will ensure a rich T'ai Chi experience for you whether you are beginning classes or a video instruction program.

Here you will discover the basic concepts of T'ai Chi, how its movements are to be performed, why they are performed that way, and how to breathe when performing them. By understanding that T'ai Chi is very different from Western exertion exercises, you won't make it harder than it is, and by relaxing into it, you unlock its full effortless potential.

T'ai Chi Posture Is Power!

You were exposed to the dan tien in Chapter 2. In T'ai Chi we move from the dan tien by first sinking into the horse stance. This is how we sink our Qi, which makes us more solid, more balanced, and more down to earth physically, emotionally, and mentally.

Make a triangle with the thumbs over the navel and forefingers extending downward. The fingertips will meet at the level of the dan tien.

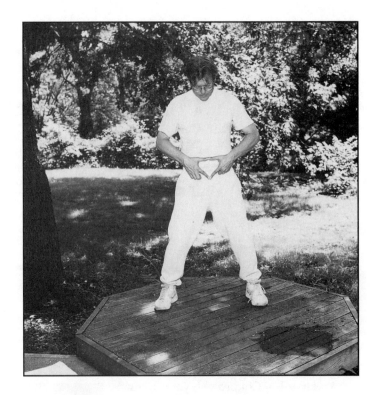

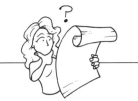

Know Your Chinese

Although the **dan tien** usually refers to an energy point below the navel, there are actually three dan tien points: one below the navel (*Qi Hai*), the second at heart level (*Shan Zhong*), and the third at eyebrow level (*Yin Tang*), all near the center of the body. Each dan tien is an energy center where certain energies are focused or supercharged into the system.

Where Is the Dan Tien?

Where the dan tien is located on the outside of the body only tells its height, for the dan tien is actually inside the body. The following will describe how to find the dan tien inside:

➤ With the fingers forming a triangle as described in the figure above, point fingers as if they could extend inside the body.

➤ Now, your fingers are pointing toward the dan tien; however, the dan tien is near the center of the body, so it can only be felt on the inside.

➤ Now tighten your sphincter muscles, as if you were pulling up your internal organs from within, and then immediately relax. Repeat this over and over, until you experience a subtle tugging sensation inside, just beyond where your fingers are pointing in to your upper pelvis or lower abdomen.

➤ That place where you feel that subtle tugging feeling is where your dan tien is. That isn't your dan tien itself—that was a muscle tugging, for your dan tien is an energy center.

➤ Dan tien can only be experienced as energy, tingling, or other light sensations. This is where all powerful movement or action comes from, and cultivated awareness of the dan tien with T'ai Chi makes any action you take more powerful, with less likelihood of injury.

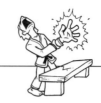

Ouch!

The lengthening of the spine that occurs as you sink into your Horse Stance is not a "forced" position. Do not "stand at attention"; rather, allow the muscles around the backbone to let go, enabling you to relax into a lengthened posture.

The Horse Stance and Dan Tien Ride Together Again

The dan tien is the basis of the Horse Stance. The Horse Stance is the basic stance for all martial arts, including T'ai Chi. It aligns the three dan tien points, *upper*, *middle*, and *lower*, to give you the best posture and most effortless movement.

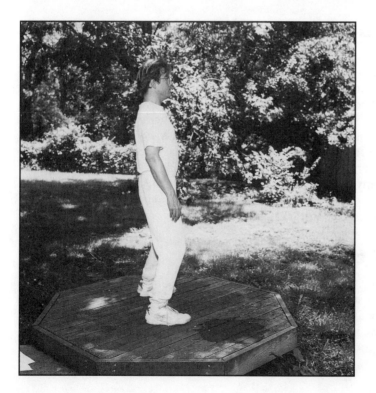

Note that the head is drawn upward toward the sky, as if a string were pulling from the center of the head. The chin is slightly pulled in, and the tailbone or sacrum is dropped down. This has the effect of lengthening the spine.

This illustrates how the spine is lengthened as you drop into the Horse Stance, although this is an exaggeration.

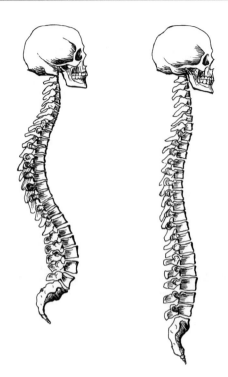

The Vertical Axis and You

Many lower back injuries are caused by poor performance posture. T'ai Chi will encourage you to maintain good posture and will remind you when you get sloppy. Proper posture is found in aligning the three dan tien points over the soles of the feet, with the weight slightly more to the heels than the front. As you practice T'ai Chi's slow gentle forms, your back will experience discomfort whenever you forget posture and let your butt creep out too much. However, the slow, low-impact nature of T'ai Chi will alert you to correct posture long before real damage occurs. This is what sets T'ai Chi apart from other training. If done correctly, slowly, and gently, T'ai Chi lets you become aware of any poor physical habits long before physical damage is done. In fact, you often don't become aware of problems in high-impact sports until the doctor is telling you not to play that sport *ever again*.

Everything and the Sinking Qi

T'ai Chi is about sinking. This isn't like heaviness as in a ship sinking, but more of a weightless release of muscles, allowing the skeleton to effortlessly hold the weight of the body. We let our relaxed shoulders sink away from our neck as we sink into our movements. It's as if we were swimming through an atmosphere of effortlessness as we move through our forms.

Sinking Your Weight

Each T'ai Chi movement is associated with an inhale and or an exhale. When we move and exhale, we allow the body to sink into a feeling of effortlessness. This is how it's done: As you transfer your weight from one leg to the other, relax the entire weight of the body down into the weight-bearing leg. The Chinese call this "sinking your Qi." By practicing this in T'ai Chi you will move more effortlessly, and your balance will improve. This also promotes blood and energy circulation through the body and encourages less joint damage by removing chronic tension from your daily movements. Tight muscles make tighter joints.

Don't Tear the Rice Paper!

In the TV series *Kung Fu*, you may have seen Kwai Chang Cane walk across the rice paper for his graduation ceremony at the Shao Lin Temple. This looked very mystical, but it was actually a very practical test.

The purpose of the test was to discover if he was pivoting the foot that was carrying his weight. In most T'ai Chi, we do not pivot the weight-bearing foot because this can destabilize our balance. More importantly, doing this can also cause knee damage. Styles that do pivot on weight-bearing legs do so rarely and take certain precautions to prevent injury. These pivots are not recommended for arthritis sufferers.

T'ai Chi movement is a process of "filling" and "emptying" each leg of Qi, or weight. The position of the dan tien over a leg determines that it is full, and the other leg is empty. We "fill" the opposite foot by shifting our dan tien over that opposite foot. Then our "empty" foot has no weight on it and can be pivoted with zero damage to the knee.

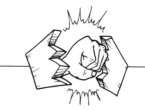

A T'ai Chi Punch Line

An advanced T'ai Chi student went to study with a grand master in China. The grand master told him to stand on one leg and said, "Keep standing, I'll be back." The grand master returned 15 minutes later and reached down to squeeze the student's calf muscle on the leg he was standing on. The master scoffed, "Too tight! Why is your leg so tight? Keep standing, I'll come back and check later."

Ouch!

There are some T'ai Chi styles that do require pivoting a weight-bearing foot. To accomplish this with no damage to the knee, you lift the dan tien at the same time so as to relieve pressure on the knee. If you have knee problems, I recommend not performing these types of pivots. But you can modify the form to be safe for you.

The vertical axis of the head and heart dan tien points lines up over the lower dan tien. This axis moving over a leg is filling that leg with Qi, or weight. As we let our breath out and relax our body weight onto a leg, we sink our Qi into that leg.

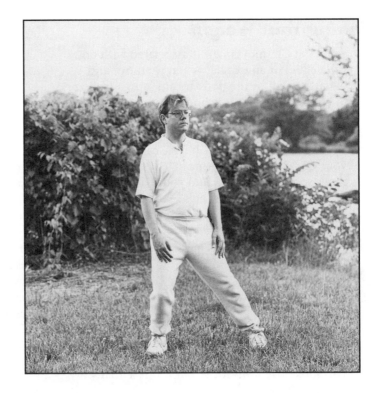

Active Bones Under Soft Muscle

T'ai Chi is unlike any exercise you have ever done because it is done best when done easily. T'ai Chi's way will also provide a model for practicing the art of effortlessness in everything we do.

T'ai Chi Is Not Isometrics

Most Western exercises involve some type of force or strain. T'ai Chi does not. The more effortlessly you are moving, the better you are doing it. You may catch yourself subconsciously tightening muscles because we have been taught that exercise must cause strain. Also, at first, your balance may not be very solid, and you will tighten your leg muscles a lot to hold you steady. This is normal, and over time, you'll find that you can relax your muscles more and more. As you get used to proper posture, using the vertical axis alignment, you'll need less muscle tension to hold you up. So, don't be discouraged if T'ai Chi doesn't feel so "effortless" at first. We are learning how to move effortlessly, by first becoming aware of how tight we are, and then by using QiGong breathing techniques you'll learn in Part 3, we begin to "let go" of needless effort as we move through T'ai Chi movements *and life.*

When doing T'ai Chi warmups, let your mind let go of thoughts, and center on your effortless breath. Then enjoy the sensations of the muscles loosening as you move. On each breath think of letting the muscles beneath the muscles let go, letting go of each other, and letting go of the bones beneath. As we relax our muscles the bones moving beneath provide a deep tissue massage, and the body can cleanse itself of toxins. Also, the relaxed abdominal muscles allow a gentle massage of the internal organs, which tonifies them and improves their function.

Don't force yourself to go as low or deep in your stances as your instructor. You have the rest of your life to get lower. Right now just focus on breathing, relaxing, and letting the muscles relax on the bones, again by allowing the entire body to relax as you exhale.

Ouch!

Becoming more comfortable with your forms and using proper posture with the vertical axis allow you to relax more as you move. At first you will notice yourself losing balance as much or even more than before you started T'ai Chi. This is not unusual. Before, you probably held your balance by holding your body tightly. Now, you are learning to balance while loose.

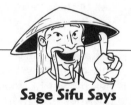

Sage Sifu Says

Don't fall into an "all or nothing" trap of self-sabotage. For example, you may have a knee problem that prevents you from rotating your knees the way the instructor does, or your asthma may prevent you from breathing as deeply or effortlessly as you would like. That's perfectly fine and natural. Do what you can in a way that feels good to you.

QiGong and T'ai Chi often help people lessen their reliance on pain or asthma medications does not mean you "must" give up your medication. On the contrary, use what works and helps you live better. Yet ironically, over time T'ai Chi and QiGong may reduce your reliance on the very medications that help you feel comfortable enough to move and breathe through T'ai Chi.

The knees are always bent in T'ai Chi. The depth of that bend depends on what feels good to you. Someone with knee problems may bend his or her knees only slightly at first, whereas someone more athletic may bend more. Do not let competitiveness cause you to go any deeper than feels good. You won't win a prize, and you'll enjoy the class less because you are straining too much. The relaxed bend of the knees allows the rest of the body to be more loose and flexible, especially the hips.

Easy Does It

Again, T'ai Chi is a mind/body exercise that integrates our mental, emotional, and physical aspects. Therefore, as you learn to move more effortlessly, you will notice that emotionally and mentally you will find ways to move through life with less and less effort. This doesn't mean you will get less done. You will probably get more done because someone with calm emotions and a relaxed mind is much more creative than someone who is in constant mental or emotional turmoil.

T'ai Sci

Some doctors believe that our central nervous system is affected by the rhythms of our breath. This means that a restriction in a freely moving respiratory system could lead to disease, since the central nervous system regulates all other organs. The goal of T'ai Chi is to foster unrestricted breathing. By doing so, T'ai Chi may improve central nervous system function, which may reduce the incidence of disease.

So, as you study T'ai Chi, be aware of patterns you may have that make learning T'ai Chi more difficult. You may find that you push yourself very hard, straining at every movement. Or you may discover that you are hypercritical of yourself, or perhaps you will sabotage your progress by avoiding practice and skipping classes. All of these patterns are probably something that you do in all aspects of your life, not just in T'ai Chi. By learning how to "play" T'ai Chi in a process of effortless learning, without strain, self-judgement, or self-sabotage, you will discover a new way to learn. By discovering a new way to learn T'ai Chi, you create a new, more effective way to learn in all your life's endeavors. You will become more successful and self actualizing by becoming clearer and more self-aware of unconscious patterns that inhibit the realization of your dreams.

Round Is Cool

In Chinese, the word for "round" is roughly equivalent to the American slang word, "cool." The Chinese felt that roundness was calming and comforting, and T'ai Chi is filled with images of roundness. We often move our hands over imaginary orbs or spheres of energy that over time become tangible enough to feel. This practice, although at first a little alien, becomes very soothing over time. It helps us become attuned to our sensations. It is like practicing "feeling." Practice makes perfect, and this is no exception.

Ouch!

Rapid expansion of the chest cavity may not efficiently oxygenate the body. However, the relaxed abdominal breathing of QiGong can be highly effective in increasing circulation of blood and Qi.

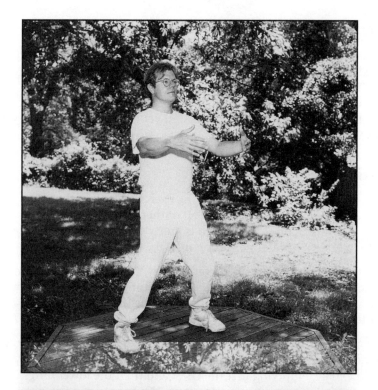

In this Moving QiGong exercise, your hands begin at groin level and circle up as if stroking a huge three-foot pearl in front of your torso. Move your hands up over and down the back of the pearl.

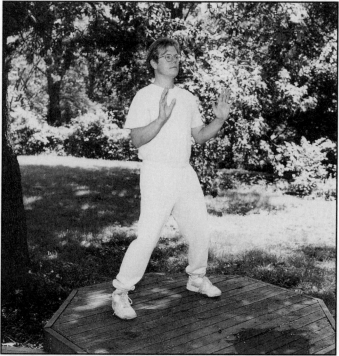

After the hands slide up and over the giant pearl, they descend along the backside until coming to rest in front of the chest, as if you were about to push someone.

Breath Is the Beginning of Everything

The essence of T'ai Chi is the breath. While doing T'ai Chi, you inhale or exhale with every movement. There is nothing more effortless in the entire universe than the release of a full breath. Therefore, T'ai Chi's ability to weave exhales with the relaxation of sinking our Qi into our weight shifts creates a powerful habit. This habit of relaxed breathing through everything we do is simple, and yet may change the way we live the rest of our lives. But again, the reason to do it is because *it feels good.*

Post-Birth Breathing

There are many QiGong breathing exercises. All QiGong exercises are breathing exercises when you get down to it. However, among all of them there are two main forms of breathing. One is *post-birth breathing*, which is pretty normal, and the second is *pre-birth breathing*, which takes a little more getting used to.

The names of these breathing forms may be based on the fact that we drew breath in through the umbilical cord prior to birth, and we draw air in through the upper body afterward. This is reflected in the way we draw air into the body during QiGong breathing, depending on which type we are doing.

With post-birth, or normal, breathing, the abdominal muscles expand out a bit as you breathe in to the abdomen, then the chest expands as the top of the lungs fills. They then relax back in as you exhale, emptying first the chest and then the lower lungs. This is how T'ai Chi and many QiGong exercises are done. However, some QiGong exercises employ pre-birth breathing.

During post-birth breathing, do not force the breath, but rather allow the body to relax as the breath enters. The following figure illustrates post-birth breathing:

Four-step post-birth breathing chart.

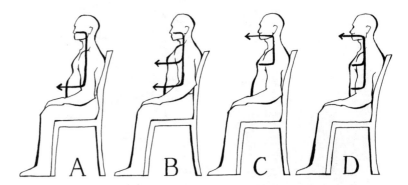

1. Breathe into the lower lungs as the abdomen relaxes slightly outward.
2. Allow the lungs and upper chest to fill as well.

3. As the body relaxes with the exhale of breath, the upper chest deflates first.

4. Then the abdomen relaxes in, completely expelling the air from the lungs.

This can be repeated for 10 or 15 minutes if you like, with wonderful results for mind and body.

Pre-Birth Breathing

Pre-birth breathing is just the opposite. As you inhale, draw the abdominal muscles in gently, and as you exhale allow them to relax. Each breathing method has different qualities and will be discussed during the moving exercises in Parts 3, 4, and 5.

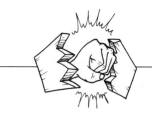

A T'ai Chi Punch Line

The Chinese believe that pre-birth breathing moves our Qi through the lower dan tien. This energy is associated with cell regeneration and sexual or procreative energy. It is therefore believed that pre-birth breathing heightens the regenerative ability of our life energy and actually slows the aging process.

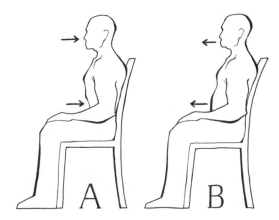

Two-step pre-birth breathing chart.

Pre-birth breathing is sort of the opposite of normal breathing. In pre-birth breathing:

1. The abdomen, especially the lower abdomen, is gently and slightly drawn in as you inhale.

2. Then, when you exhale, the abdomen relaxes back out.

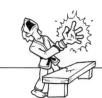

Ouch!

Pre-birth breathing involves a bit of training and some cautionary notes. It is advisable to practice normal post-birth breathing only during your exercises, unless training with an experienced QiGong instructor.

The Least You Need to Know

➤ Your posture is your power.

➤ Sinking Qi improves your balance.

➤ T'ai Chi practice protects your joints.

➤ Proper breath techniques are the most powerful health tool.

Part 3

Starting Down the QiGong Path to T'ai Chi

Part 3 details how QiGong can lubricate the way for us to fit into a new world developing around us in these rapidly changing times. Practical exercises for young, old, and everyone in between will help you breathe the breath of life and have some fun doing it. Here you will also learn some QiGong history and see why some QiGong is different than T'ai Chi. Learning QiGong will make your T'ai Chi experience much richer. It is said that medicine cures, but the best medicine prevents. Chapter 10 will discuss not only the personal healing powers of QiGong, but how you can share your Qi, or life energy, with others. Part 3 will alert you to some common challenges you may encounter as you begin exploring your inner self with Sitting QiGong. Then, the Sitting QiGong exercise presented in Chapter 11 will get your Qi overflowing. In fact it will lead you through an explanation and exercise that may actually change the way you view the universe you live in. Chapter 12 exposes you to the beautiful and wonderful feeling of Moving QiGong exercises, or Dong Gong. There are thousands of them, so in this chapter you will only be able to dip your toe into an ocean of what's out there. The T'ai Chi warmup exercises detailed in Chapter 13 are QiGong exercises that not only calm the mind, but prepare the body for T'ai Chi. These exercises alone can have a wonderful impact on your day.

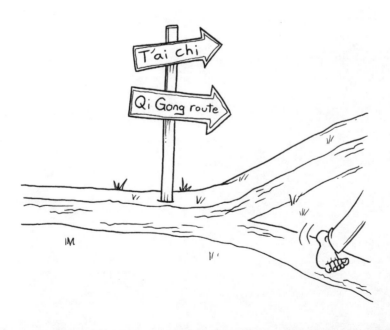

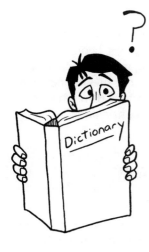

Chapter 10

What Is QiGong?

In This Chapter

➤ Learn why breathing is so important

➤ How QiGong and T'ai Chi differ

➤ Why QiGong is beyond meditation

➤ QiGong is medicine

➤ Survive and flourish through QiGong challenges

➤ External QiGong heals others

The purpose of QiGong is to let go of energy blocks by relaxing the mind, body, and emotions. Although T'ai Chi shares this purpose, there are QiGong exercises that are not T'ai Chi.

QiGong differs from standard meditations but shares many of their healing potentials. QiGong can be used as therapy for specific conditions, as well as a general tune up. Also, we can actually treat another person with the life energy QiGong fills us with.

Also, there are different types of QiGong. There is active QiGong (Dong Gong) and passive QiGong (Jing Gong). Active QiGong involves obvious movement, like T'ai Chi. Passive is where the external body is still but the awareness is directed and felt in various areas of the body, by breath, or imagery, or both.

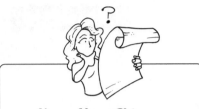

We encounter many challenges when beginning QiGong practice. By realizing that these are common, you can begin to move past them and get all the benefits QiGong offers. These challenges to QiGong practice represent challenges we face in all aspects of our life and personal growth. Therefore, by learning to move through these challenges in QiGong, we begin to untie knots in many other parts of our lives as well.

Know Your Chinese

Literally translated, **Qi** means "air," or "energy" and **gong** means "work." Therefore, QiGong literally translated means "Breath Work," or "Energy Work."

Let's Do Some Heavy Breathing

Many ancient cultures have recognized the breath as our connection with the life force, or Qi. In Chinese, the character for Qi, or life energy, is the same character used for air, as in breath. In Latin, the *"spir"* of *spir*it or re*spir*ate, means "to breathe." Spirit is the *breath of life,* or life energy, which is another word for Qi. So, in both the East and West, breath was recognized as the key to life's energy. To breathe shallowly therefore means that you are cheating yourself out of a lot of life.

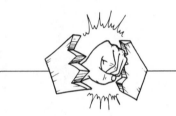

Don't Be T'ai Shy

Many T'ai Chi classes begin with Sitting QiGong exercises that require us to breathe deeply. You may find this difficult because our lungs have lost capacity from lack of use, or our back and chest muscles are tight with tension. This will change. As your rigid muscles relax, you will soon discover your lungs finding new capacity.

Some are just embarrassed to let other people hear us breathe. Maybe it's because we only think of hearing deep breathing during sex or other intense feelings, and we're taught not to show our feelings in public. After a few classes, people get more comfortable with each other and get comfortable with the idea of breathing. Then the tentative group transforms into *a wild bunch of breathing bohemians!*

A T'ai Chi Punch Line

A corporate executive arriving promptly for a QiGong class informed the instructor, "My doctor said QiGong would be good for my heart condition, so I want to learn QiGong. But I heard about all that weird breathing you do. I want you to know, I am not into the breathing thing." The instructor responded, "We'd better hurry and get you into it before it's too late because I don't do CPR."

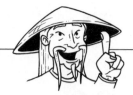

Sage Sifu Says

If you forget everything about QiGong except to remember to breathe deeply when under stress, you will find great benefit. Of course, that is only the beginning—the key to the door of what T'ai Chi has to offer—so don't stop there.

Yawning Is Believing—in Yourself

So QiGong first of all teaches us to feel good about ourselves and to follow what our body wants and needs, like breathing deeply, *even in public*. In fact, QiGong practitioners get to where they can even yawn in public. I know that may seem pretty risqué now, but after learning QiGong, even you will be able to yawn unashamedly in public. And this ability will reflect an even deeper ability to believe in yourself enough to do what your body tells you it needs, whether it's more rest, better foods, regular gentle exercise, or a good solid yawn, even in the middle of a department meeting.

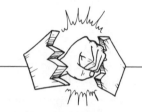

A T'ai Chi Punch Line

A Chinese T'ai Chi master was asked, "Why do we do T'ai Chi?" His answer was, "To burp." He meant that T'ai Chi makes us aware of what the body needs and self-assured enough to satisfy those healthful needs. A yawn is a form of deep release, both physical and mental. To deny that release is not a healthy habit. Yawn away!

T'ai Chi vs. QiGong: What's the Diff?

T'ai Chi's goal of relaxing the mind and body to encourage the flow of energy through us makes it QiGong. However, not all QiGong is T'ai Chi (because some QiGong is sitting or lying, and all T'ai Chi is moving and standing). The mental strain of trying to figure whether you are doing T'ai Chi or QiGong will limit your ability to get the benefits. Forget about it. As you practice T'ai Chi and QiGong exercises, the differences will become obvious.

Don't sweat it; after Parts 3 and 4, you'll be an expert on the tenets of both T'ai Chi and QiGong. Remember, much of T'ai Chi and QiGong are interchangeable and synonymous anyway. As stated before, the premise of all Traditional Chinese Medicine, of which T'ai Chi and QiGong are integral parts, is that energy flows through the

T'ai Sci

In the Chinese Medica there are about 7,000 different breathing exercises, all gentle, all pleasant, and all QiGong. In Traditional Chinese hospitals, physicians may prescribe a QiGong exercise to help heal a problem, much the same way that a Western doctor might prescribe a drug (of course QiGong exercises only have *good* side effects). Many Western doctors are now beginning to prescribe T'ai Chi and QiGong as well.

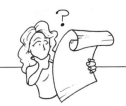

Know Your Chinese

The *Taoist Canon* (1145 AD) held all the early writing on QiGong, although at that time it was known as Tao-yin. QiGong is a fairly modern term. Taoist philosophy emphasizes being attuned to the invisible laws of nature. QiGong, or Tao-yin, was viewed as a way to connect with that deeper part of ourselves that knows what is best for us.

body, and we are likely to get sick when it gets blocked off. So QiGong's goal to allow the mind and body to release the past and fears of the future in order to live a more flowing, healthful life is also the goal of T'ai Chi.

QiGong and Other Meditations

QiGong is a form of meditation; however, it can be more as well. QiGong can actively be used to treat a specific organ or an area of pain and discomfort by directing Qi to that area.

Like other meditations, such as za-zen or transcendental meditation, QiGong allows the mind to empty of active thought and be passively aware. In za-zen this state of mind is achieved by not thinking about anything, but just letting thoughts drift through the mind without fixing or holding onto them. In transcendental meditation, a *mantra* (a verbal utterance used in meditation), or perhaps a *mandala* (a visual meditation tool), is used to take the mind out of the problem-solving mode and into a state of free flow, whereby it "observes" rather than "thinks about" things that flow through the mind.

QiGong combines this passive awareness, or "letting go," with an active healing intention. If treating a headache, for example, once we think about the energy filling the muscles in our head, we have to let that thought go and then just experience how nice it feels as Qi's healing energy, or light relaxes the head. We observe the healing release in the tight muscles, and, in a way, the passive observation of our own healing becomes a mantra or mandala.

History of QiGong: Welcome Back to the Future!

QiGong is believed to be over 2,000 years old. Its roots are with ancient Chinese farmers who observed that nature's balance makes things strong. Moderation, flexibility, and constant nurturing filled crops with the life force, or Qi. These ancient observers developed exercises that mimicked that healthy way of cultivating life energy.

Back to the Future

What many Western hospitals are now treating as cutting-edge treatments for cancer, for example, can be found in the 800-year-old *Taoist Canon*. At the Simonton Cancer Center, mental imagery exercises are successfully used to help cancer sufferers live nearly twice as long as their peers who do not use imagery techniques. The *Taoist Canon* wrote of thousands of visualization techniques meant to heal various conditions.

So the world has come full circle and what was ancient treatment in China is now the cutting edge of modern healing in the West. *Welcome back to the future.*

Is Your Mind Half Full or Half Empty?

Here in the West, we have no trouble understanding and accepting that our mind can make us sick. We know that worry can cause an ulcer or that chronic anxiety can lead to a heart attack. However, we have a big problem accepting just the opposite, that our mind can also heal us.

It's an "is the glass half full or half empty" kind of thing. We know that our stress can cause our shoulders to tighten and our breath to get shallow and constricted, leading to hypertension and maybe a headache. But the concept of using our mind to heal us is thought of as a "weird" idea. Ponder this: We all know that recalling an argument we had a week ago or even a month ago can cause our muscles to tighten, our breathing to shallow, and our blood pressure to skyrocket. *Now, that is strange!*

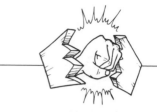

A T'ai Chi Punch Line

The ultimate source of Chinese medical knowledge is The Yellow Emperor's *Classic of Internal Medicine* (200 BC), which prescribed QiGong for curing and preventing illness. According to this ancient book, true medicine cured diseases before they developed. T'ai Chi and QiGong can be very effective at doing just that.

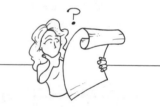

Know Your Chinese

QiGong has had other names in the past, such as *tu gu na xin*, "expelling the old energy, absorbing the new," or *tao-yin*, "leading and guiding the energy." Actually, the term QiGong is a fairly recent way of saying energy exercise.

So, if something as abstract as a week-old memory can wreak havoc on our health, it makes perfect sense that our mind can have a healing effect on itself today. Unlocking its grip on worry and tension, the mind can allow each cell to bathe in the radiant glow of health.

Boredom? It's QiGong Time!

T'ai Sci

Western medical research has discovered that our immune system follows certain rhythms; that it is weakest at about 1 a.m. and strongest at about 7 a.m. This may partially explain why when you are sick, your cold or flu symptoms keep you from sleeping at night, and then suddenly in the morning you are ready to sleep well. Ancient Chinese doctors were not only aware of this general pattern but also began to distinguish similar cycles in specific organs.

If you are wondering when to do Qigong, the short answer is, anytime you need it. In fact, as you practice energy work more and more, you will find that you always do it, in a way. As you open more to the feeling of energy flowing, rather than being squeezed off by stress, you will automatically sit back and breathe yourself open each time stress begins to close off your flow of Qi.

I always remind students that after learning QiGong, they need never again be bored. Anytime you catch yourself getting anxious in a line or in a waiting room, you now can just mentally kick back and practice these wonderful exercises instead of stressing out.

Although you can practice QiGong with great results at any time of the day, Traditional Chinese Medicine has found that the energy flowing through your body is different at different times of the day. Just as Chapter 7 explained how T'ai Chi can be performed at different times of the day for different effects, so can other QiGong exercises. Refer to Chapter 7 to see the times and related organ systems.

Mental Healing and QiGong Challenges

QiGong helps heal us mentally, emotionally, and physically, but the beginning of healing entails *becoming more aware*. This can present challenges for the novice because when we become more aware of our mental, emotional, and physical discomforts, we often think this means T'ai Chi and/or QiGong don't work. Many of us think a mind/body exercise like T'ai Chi means "instant and permanent nirvana," and when we discover that we have to "feel" discomfort such as tension before we know to let it go, we may mistakenly think the tools "don't work." Remember that this new self-awareness is part of a healing process, and you will get enormous benefits from your practice if you stick with it.

Bliss vs. Discomfort

T'ai Chi, QiGong, and other mind/body fitness exercises are sometimes mistakenly seen as "escapist," whereby we can use them to run away from our problems. Although T'ai Chi and QiGong can seem like a soothing vacation from our problems sometimes, they also help us heal or release the source of those problems.

For example, when doing Sitting QiGong exercises or meditations, you may feel your shoulders getting very tense. Remember the exercise is not making you tense. The exercise of sitting mindfulness is helping you become aware of a pattern or habit you have of holding tension in your shoulders. Now that you are aware of it, you can practice the release and relaxation systems presented in Chapter 11 to begin to let that pattern go.

As you practice T'ai Chi and/or QiGong, you may experience tension or even anxiety. Do not let that stop you or make you think you are doing it wrong. The emergence of these feelings is an opportunity to begin releasing them, using your new tools of breath and life energy.

Trying Too Hard to See the Light?

If your QiGong exercises make you feel intensely anxious or tense, it's usually because you are trying too hard to make the tools work. Ironically, the harder we try to relax, let go, and make light or life energy flow through us, the more we squeeze it off.

Life energy flows effortlessly through us when we let the mind and body let go. This is what QiGong teaches us to do. Furthermore, QiGong practice will teach you how to let your conscious mind work with the effortless power of life energy. This will take practice. You will catch yourself trying too hard to feel life energy or trying too hard to make muscles relax. Always remember that the Qi, or life energy, is completely effortless. Your mind or thoughts can direct your Qi to tense shoulder muscles, but once that thought is directed, you can and must let your mind relax, letting go of the outcome.

Chi, I'm a Healer!?! External QiGong

That's right, you are a healer, master. After practicing the Sitting QiGong exercise in Chapter 11, you will feel the Qi flowing out of your hands. Medical studies have shown that this energy can help people heal. Most nursing schools in the United States now teach a form of External QiGong called Therapeutic Touch and are finding great success with everything from anxiety reduction to facilitating healing. If someone you know has a headache, you can usually get some results even if you are a novice. Whether you completely heal the headache or not, he will likely get some relief, or at the very least, his headache won't last as long as it normally would.

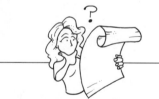

Know Your Chinese

Wai Qi Zhi Liao is the term for External QiGong. Modern Therapeutic Touch used in many Western hospitals is a form of External QiGong.

In the following figures, you will see one form of an External QiGong exercise you can begin practicing today. After completing steps 1, 2, and 3, ask the recipient to describe to you how he or she feels, before proceeding to step 4. Your experience with these tools is the best teacher of what they offer you and others.

The giver of energy stands to one side of the receiver, with his hands extended over the recipient's heart.

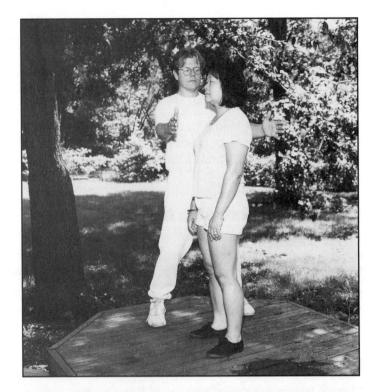

Then he slowly brings his hands over the recipient's shoulder and down her arm to allow the giver's Qi to flow from his hands into the recipient's arm.

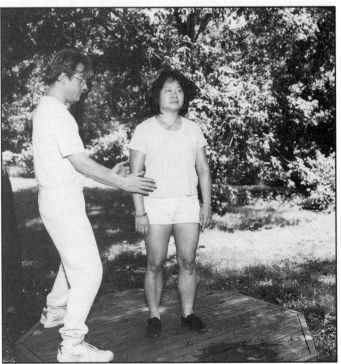

1. As you let your Qi flow through your hands into the receiver's heart, slowly bring your hands over her shoulder and down, keeping the receiver's arm between your hands so your Qi can flow into her arm.

2. Bring your hands back up to the heart and repeat three times.

3. Shake off your hands between each brushdown to let go of any stress or heavy energy you might have brushed off on the receiver.

4. Repeat this entire process after moving to the other side, so the recipient's left and right side are both brushed down.

There are many other healing exercises for various purposes. These are general cleansing treatments that will benefit anybody. However, the recipients have to feel comfortable with the process because if they feel tense, it won't work as well. Many nurses simply place their hands on patients to comfort them and then let their energy flow into the patients without their conscious awareness of it. This allows the patients to relax.

The Least You Need to Know

➤ If you breathe, the rest is easy. *All of it.*

➤ T'ai Chi is QiGong.

➤ QiGong is an ancient/modern healing art.

➤ Discomfort is information, not an enemy.

➤ You are a healer, master.

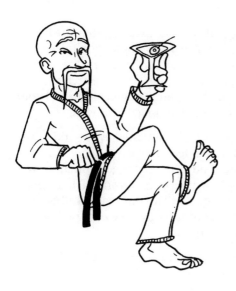

Sitting QiGong (Jing Gong)

In This Chapter

➤ Qi can be seen and felt

➤ Understanding we are only energy

➤ Sitting QiGong lights you up

➤ QiGong exercises to constantly release your stress

There are many ways to measure the Qi flowing through our bodies. A common way to see energy flow is through Kirlian photography. Chapter 11 will give you some examples of how Kirlian photography captures images of our energy.

QiGong practice isn't about pretending to be energy; it is about feeling what we really are, which is energy. Actually the entire universe is energy. This chapter ends with an exercise of Sitting QiGong, which will allow you to actually feel the nature of your energy, and how life energy, or Qi, feels as it flows through your body. You'll love it!

Energy Medicine and QiGong

Previous chapters explained how Chinese Medicine works by unblocking or directing the energy flowing through the body. QiGong and T'ai Chi also work to balance and unblock that energy.

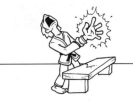

Ouch!

Some studies identify cynicism as our greatest health risk. This is because being constantly suspicious of the world around you triggers unhealthy stress responses. Keep an open mind and relaxed body as you learn about your energetic nature.

However, QiGong is also about realizing that the body isn't a solid thing, but instead an open, moving wave of energy. QiGong will actually help you realize your energy nature by providing quiet sitting exercises that enable you to feel it. Over time you'll begin to feel your energy aspect in your T'ai Chi practice as well.

The Sitting QiGong exercise presented at the end of this chapter will allow you to feel the Qi or energy that moves through your body. Before we get to that, however, let's examine how the process works. Then, when you do the exercise, you can let your brain, and skepticism, relax and get out of the way. The energy flows easier when we are *effortless*.

So don't worry about memorizing any of these facts. Rather, sit back and be entertained by the fascinating insights into who you really are.

Kirlian Photography: Seeing Qi Is Believing

There is actually a way to take photographs of the energy aspect of our body. You may have heard this energy referred to as auras. Kirlian photography has been around since the 1950s, but it got a lot more attention as we learned about Qi and QiGong in the West. This is because Kirlian photography seems to be able to take pictures of Qi, or at least aspects of Qi.

When a Kirlian photograph is taken, the person, or leaf, or any living thing, rests on a photographic plate, and a mild electrical current is run through it. Then the camera takes an image of the energy or Qi of the plant or person.

Phantom of the Aura

When Kirlian photography was first introduced, skeptics argued that the photography captured nothing more than the electricity running through the plant or person's hand or whatever was photographed. However, this all changed with the discovery of the "phantom effect." The following figure illustrates the phantom effect, seen on a leaf.

In these front and back images, you see a leaf, but what's amazing is that the top part of the leaf that you see *isn't there!* The top quarter of the leaf has been torn off. So, what looks like a leaf is actually the Qi, or energy aspect, of the top of the leaf. You can see where the leaf was torn, but still see the veins and edges of the leaf going up. This discovery changed not only the way people viewed Kirlian photography, *but also the way science began to look at what we are made of.*

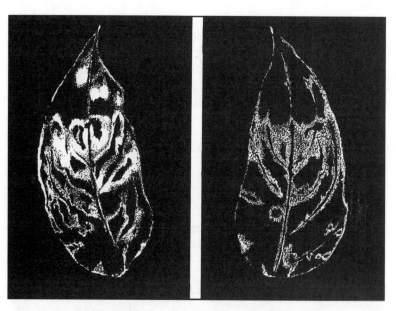

This illustration represents the "phantom effect" as it appears in a common Kirlian photograph of a leaf.

The T'ai Chi Zone, Do-Do-Do-Do, Do-Do-Do-Do

The following figure illustrates how our behavior affects our Qi or energy. This is important for understanding the benefits of the Sitting QiGong exercise we will do later. Eating right, getting enough rest and exercise, and practicing T'ai Chi and QiGong can positively affect your energy flow, whereas behavior shown to be detrimental to health can negatively affect Qi flow.

The following figure shows a woman's fingertip and the energy flowing through and around it. The image on the left shows this woman's fingertip in a normal state. The Chinese would call that Smooth Qi, or a healthful state. However, the image to the right is the same woman after she drank a cup of coffee and smoked her very first cigarette. The energy went wild! In fact, notice that in some places, there seems to be no energy.

We all know how smooth Qi feels, as on those days when you wake up and everything just clicks the way it's supposed to. Every paper wad you throw lands right in the center of the trash can. In basketball, they call it being *in the zone*. So we all know how it feels when we are there, in the zone, but we might not know how to get there.

T'ai Sci

An excellent book, *The Tao of Physics* (listed in the back of this book), shows how the modern subatomic physicists' view of reality is often very close to the view held by ancient Chinese mystics. By going within themselves in QiGong meditation, these mystics somehow began to understand what modern physics understands about the energetic nature of reality.

Kirlian photographs illustrate how our behavior affects our energy flow or Qi flow through our body and beyond.

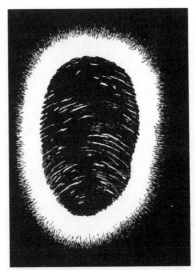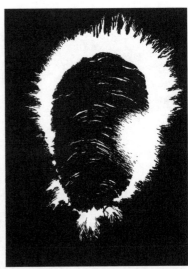

What T'ai Chi and QiGong offer is a way to get into the zone. As we practice our T'ai Chi movements every day, day after day, we find ourselves spending much less time frazzled and wired, like in the second image. And we find ourselves more and more in the calm center of Smooth Qi, like in the first image.

Mind Over Qi

The following figure is very important in preparing you for the upcoming Sitting QiGong exercise because it illustrates how our minds can direct energy. In this figure you see two sets of hands, both belong to the same man. In the image on the left, you see his hands in a normal state. However, in the image on the right, you see his hands when he's consciously thinking of *sending energy* out through his hands.

When the man was thinking of *sending energy* out of his hands, he wasn't grunting and straining. He simply relaxed as he *let it happen.* I mention this before you start the Sitting QiGong to it remind you not to "try."

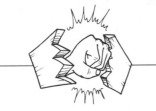

A T'ai Chi Punch Line

Twenty years ago, I smoked about two packs a day. It was nearly impossible for me to sit still for 20 minutes to do Sitting Qigong—because in Sitting QiGong we begin to become conscious of the energy disruption our habits cause. However, over time as my energy flowed more smoothly, I scaled back on my smoking and eventually replaced the need for cigarettes with the pleasure of my renewed energy flow.

This is an important point because we often think that anything worth doing must be hard. We want to put our "shoulder to the wheel," our "nose to the grindstone," "furrowing the brow" to get something done. However, the energy work, or QiGong, doesn't work that way. The more you try, the more the muscles tighten up, and the less the energy flows through you.

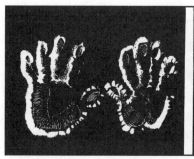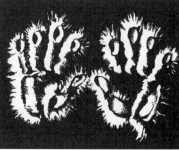

Kirlian photographs illustrate how our energy or Qi flow can be directed by thought.

So, as the man (illustrated in the above figure) was sending energy out his hands, he just thought of it happening, and then relaxed and enjoyed the feeling as he let it flow out. You may experience what he felt during the Sitting QiGong exercise.

The Sitting QiGong is a very effortless process. When it begins, I'll invoke images, such as a soothing flow of relaxation or light energy pouring over your head and face, relaxing all the muscles. When you read this or hear it on an audiotape (you may find it helpful to record the Sitting QiGong in your voice and then listen with your eyes closed rather than reading), you will want to imagine the shower of lightness or relaxation pouring over you. But then let go of the image and just enjoy the feeling of effortless relaxation spreading through your head and facial muscles as the lightness spreads through them.

In research it is found that if you think of the image, let go of that mental image, and then let the lightness flow through, you will be more able to feel the pleasure of that flow.

T'ai Sci

Harvard Medical School did studies on several relaxation response techniques and found that one thing is necessary to get the most out of any of the exercises. You have to adopt a state of mind called "passive awareness" or "effortless concentration." This means that you can't force the experience of QiGong.

E=mc2 Means You are Only Energy

It's easier to relax and let your Qi flow through you if you know that everything in the universe is only made out of energy, *including you*. Einstein's famous equation $E=mc^2$ means, E (energy) equals m (mass) times c (speed of light squared). Don't get an algebra attack though, again because all it means is that all things, including you, are made of energy.

Actually, we are mostly just empty space. To understand just how spacious we all are consider the following. If you could take an atom out of anything in the universe, like one of your body's atoms, and blow it up to the size of a football field, the nucleus of that atom would only be the size of a BB in the center of that football field. The

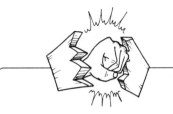

A T'ai Chi Punch Line

In a T'ai Chi class at a senior center in Kansas, a feisty 95-year old woman missed the first class and had to be caught up. She nodded, listening very attentively as I explained how we are all made of energy, and then I asked her "What do you think?" She replied, "Sonny, you've got a vivid imagination!"

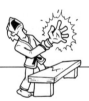

Ouch!

Don't feel as though you have to sit perfectly still while doing the Sitting QiGong exercise. If you need to fidget, roll out your neck or shoulders, scratch an itch, or yawn constantly, let yourself do it. Let your body be as loose and comfortable as possible. However, don't let your mind be distracted by having your eyes open. Close your eyes after reading each point, giving yourself time to experience the effects of each suggestion.

electrons that revolve around it would be like dust motes 50 yards away in the end zone. So everything between the BB and the dust mote 50 yards away is energy field, or empty space.

In fact, imagine if you could take all the atoms of *all the human beings on the whole planet* and somehow smush all their atomic particles together, getting rid of the empty space or energy fields we are made of. All the humans on the entire planet's smushed up atomic particles would add up to just one grain of rice. That is it!

The best image to illustrate that we are mostly open, permeable space is found in something called a "particle chamber," which can be seen in children's science museums. A particle chamber is a big glass box filled with ammonia mist. The plaque on the chamber explains that there are cosmic particles falling through space, through the roof of the building, through your skull, your body, your shoes, and right into the earth as you sit here reading this. However, the particles are too small to be seen with your eyes. So the chamber's ammonia mist wraps layers of ammonia around the particles and shines bright flood lights on them, making them big enough to see. When you look inside the particle chamber, what you see is a blizzard of these particles. The same blizzard that is flowing through us all the time.

I mention all this to set the mood for the Sitting QiGong exercise. Because it reminds us that we are not solid impenetrable mass. We are mostly empty space, and the Qi or life energy can flow through our skull and brain just as easily as it flows through the air around us.

The only thing that can limit the Qi flow is a thought limitation. So, if when I invoke an image of a relaxing flow of energy pouring through your head, you think, "Hold on there, my head is solid mass," you're muscles will tighten up a bit. This tightening will restrict the flow of energy that flows through you.

QiGong and T'ai Chi do not make energy flow through you. The energy flows through you every moment that you are alive. Yet as we age, we often squeeze off the flow of life energy, turning it into a dribble, rather than the river of life that flowed through us as kids. So, T'ai Chi and QiGong work by allowing the mind and body to let go of fears, tensions, and grudges that squeeze off our energy flow. This Sitting QiGong exercise is about letting go effortlessly with every breath. The energy flows by itself.

Sitting QiGong (Jing Gong) Introduction

In this exercise you will begin to feel your flow of Qi, or life energy. The Qi will be referred to as "light" because the Qi flows right through you, like sunlight seems to soak right into your bones on a nice spring day.

Remember not to try. You are not *supposed* to see or feel anything. We are just going to have a nice relaxing experience. So, as I offer images to your mind, read them and then close your eyes and let yourself feel the result. You may want to tape record yourself reading this exercise, and then you can do it with your eyes closed. Also, you will find energy work audio tapes available for mail order in the back of this book that will guide you through this exercise.

Sage Sifu Says

To get better results and enjoy a wonderful experience, complete this exercise from beginning to end all in one sitting. This may take about 20 minutes. To only read this is not enough to understand Sitting QiGong. You must let your mind and body go through the different levels of relaxation to actually "feel" the results. Otherwise it would be like only reading about water and having never felt water.

The Qi will move through you with no effort; the words below only initiate the process, then you can sit back and enjoy as the light or Qi moves to where your thought effortlessly directs it.

A Sitting QiGong Exercise

The following exercise is best done sitting upright in a comfortable chair that supports good posture. Your feet should be in solid contact with the floor. Also, if your arms and legs are not crossed the energy flows easier. When you see spaces between text divided by ... (an ellipsis) give yourself a few seconds to assimilate and feel the experience before reading on.

1. Begin by placing your feet flat on the floor, with your palms flat on your legs. Let your eyes close comfortably and naturally. This exercise will be broken into sections so that you can open your eyes to read a section and then close them for a few moments to let yourself experience, or feel, the responses.

2. All T'ai Chi or QiGong exercises begin by simply becoming aware of the breath. Notice how your lungs fill and empty. Let your chest and back relax so that your lungs can fill from the bottom all the way up to the top of the lungs. Notice how as you release the breath, your lungs empty from the top, or the chest, and then empty all the way down into the abdomen, as the abdominal muscles pull in slightly.

Sit with feet flat, palms flat on thighs, and your back straight but not rigid.

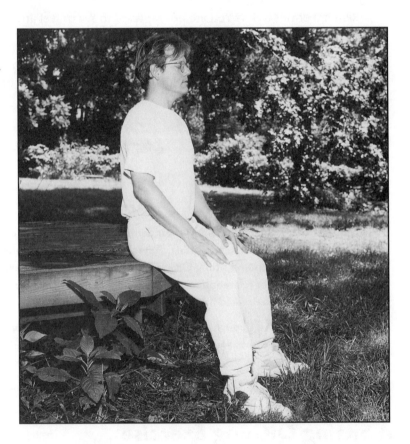

3. Let your mind relax as the muscles in your head, neck, shoulders, chest, and back relax. As the body relaxes, the breaths become not only deeper but also more effortless. Allow your awareness to relax and ride on the rhythm of that breath, as if the whole body was being breathed by the air. Let the whole body relax as you release each breath.

4. As you feel the body let go of the breath, feel the brain let go of your thoughts and worries of the day. Just as the deep exhales or releasing yawns allow the muscles to let go, the exhaled breath can also let go of mental tensions. The muscles within and around your heart likewise can hold onto fears or emotions. So as you release each breath, yawn, or sigh, allow the heart to release emotions, the body to release the muscles, and the mind to let go of worries. Each breath is a deep letting go on all levels.

5. Notice that as you let each breath out, it feels as though the atoms of the body are actually expanding away from one another. That's because they are. When we get tense, the body's atoms actually squeeze together, tightening us up. So, as we breathe and allow the body to open, the atoms and cells relax away from one another . . . feeling as if the wind could blow right through you.

6. Now, think of the sun directly above your head. Just by thinking of an orb of lightness above your head, you may experience a subtle lift or lightening throughout your mind, or your presence. This Qi, light, or subtle energy, vibrates at a higher, more silken rate than the body's vibratory rate. Therefore, you may experience a feeling of lightness, or loosening, and a deep letting go throughout your entire being. Good.

7. Let that sun open and release a shower of clear, washing light, or silken energy, to pour over your head, body, and through your feet down into the earth below. Let go of that image and open to the feeling of deep release as you are washed by that silken energy. Like a water hose spraying through a screen door, just let the body open and be washed through, as you release each sighing exhale.

Ouch!

Whenever you notice that your breathing is very shallow or that you are holding your breath, make it a point to breathe deeply. Let the body relax open, allowing air down into the bottom of the abdominal region of the lungs, and let the whole body relax that breath out, as if the breath were breathing you. Do not force, just let.

8. Be aware as a feeling of lightness expands through the tissues of the body. Notice the light spreading through the muscles in the top of your head. As the cranial muscles relax, they release their grip on the skull, allowing that permeating lightness to expand through the scalp. Expanding through the sides and back of the head, the entire scalp is lighted, as light flows out through every follicle and every hair on the head. Feel the scalp relaxing around the root of every hair.

9. Now allow the light to expand into the muscles at the base of the neck, then down and throughout the connected muscles in the shoulders and upper back. As they let go of their grip on the bones, experience the airy lightness permeating between muscles and bones . . . a deep letting go.

10. Feel as the energy expands up the back of the head and over the sides . . . feel the hinges of the jaw relax.

11. Now, allow this energy to expand over the forehead, the brow, down the bridge of the nose, and into the temples. Don't try to feel anything or make anything happen; just effortlessly observe as the light expands into the left eye socket . . . and then the right. Experience all the tiny optical muscles letting go.

12. Perceive the illumination expanding through all the soft tissue of the face, nose, mouth, and lips.

13. Experience an airy radiance expanding up through the nose into the deepest recesses of the sinus cavity. Feel that opening release as the sinuses fill with light.

14. Now, into the ears: Feel the deep skeletal muscles in the sides of the head let go as the silken energy expands into the inner ears, allowing a deep letting go in the sides of the head.

15. As the inner ears relax, the Eustachian tubes open, allowing the soothing energy to flow down into the mouth. As the mouth fills with light, the upper palate, upper jaw, gums, and even teeth seem to lighten, loosen, and let go. And now the lower jaw.

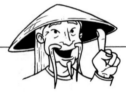

Sage Sifu Says

Do not rush through this. Be sure to close your eyes between each instruction point, allowing yourself to sit back and savor the experience of each image. Don't rush through it. Enjoy. Breathe. Breathe.

16. As you become aware of any saliva gathered in your mouth, swallow it, and experience the energy expanding down your throat, through the neck, and into your chest, shoulders, and back.

17. The heart itself can begin to lighten. If you catch yourself trying to feel or make something happen, let all that go. Be willing to feel absolutely nothing as you passively observe the lightness expanding through your heart and chest, permeating all the fibrous tissues of your lungs.

18. This allows every beat of the heart to carry lighted oxygen to all the extremities of the body; in fact, every cell begins to be lighted as the energy moves through the liquid systems of the body. Let the body open to that lightness, even in the tightest places.

19. Allow the light to expand through the abdomen, lighting the stomach . . . the liver . . . intestinal tract . . . kidneys . . . and lower back.

20. Now, think of the sun above your head again. Think of it opening and releasing an even greater flow of light over and through the body. Once you think the thought, let go of it, and experience the feeling of expanded release . . . as the bones themselves begin to lighten, the deepest skeletal muscles begin to release their grip on the bones.

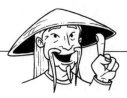

Sage Sifu Says

The light or Qi heals and lifts without any effort on your part; let go of those tight head muscles and enjoy the feeling of release.

21. As the skull becomes permeated with light, the soothing energy expands right into the brain, illuminating the left frontal lobe and then the right frontal lobe, and expanding into the forebrain, above and just behind the eyes, into the midbrain and temporal lobes, and on into the brainstem, or old brain, in back.

22. Experience as all the billions of brain cells open up to that silken effortless radiance. It's as if the brain were a muscle that we've held clenched very tightly for a long, long time. And now as we allow the light to expand through the brain, we are finally allowing that muscle to let go, to expand open, and to light.

23. Now let the energy expand through the spine to the entire nervous system. Any nervous tension on the frayed nerve endings can now be released into that silken healing lightness now passing through all the nerves to the furthest dendrites in the skin.

24. Experience the light flowing down to the tip of the tail bone and radiating out, filling the pelvic bowl, and expanding on down through the legs and feet. Now think of the feet opening to allow this river of cleansing energy to pour right through into the cleansing pull of the earth.

25. Let the whole body open to be washed through as the feet release any loads or heavy tensions down into the earth's cleansing pull.

26. As you allow yourself to be washed through by this radiant cleansing shower, you may become aware of blocks in the flow. Tight spots, tensions, anxiety, feelings of restlessness, or thick drowsiness may appear. Any discomfort you feel is due to a block in the flow of energy. Note where you may feel those blocks or discomforts. Take a deep breath, and as you close your eyes, let the breath out. Think of the light expanding in the center of that tightness or blockage. Experience the opening release.

27. This enables the light to expand in the center of the blockage, allowing that area to open up. Release the blockage into the cleansing shower that pours through you to wash the blockage away and release it out through the feet into the earth. Breathe and release yet a bit deeper with every exhale, as if the bones themselves could let go of the load they carry.

28. Sit in this cleansing downpour for a while, enjoying the release. As any thoughts, worries, or tensions surface in your mind or heart, release them into the cleansing shower of washing light. Breathe, release, and enjoy.

29. Now, think of the feet closing. Instantly that happens, with no effort. By closing the feet, you may experience a sensation of back-filling energy on the soles of your feet as the light fills the feet and the field around, like a silken cocoon of light, coming up over the feet, ankles, knees, legs, and torso, and spilling over the top of your head to fill the field around you.

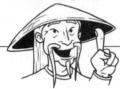

Sage Sifu Says

Our thought directs energy, and once directed, it moves there without any effort on our part. Having our eyes closed allows us to experience this within ourselves, to enjoy the cleansing release. This is effortless. The light or Qi, moves with no effort. Once you think the thought, let it go, and sit back and enjoy responses.

30. With the eyes closed, lift your hands in front of you, as if you were holding a giant beach ball between your palms (see the following figure). Think of the palms and fingers opening, and effortlessly the back-filling energy in your body now flows out through your palms and fingers.

31. Take a few deep-cleansing breaths to release all the muscles in your upper body, even though your hands are raised. It's the letting go that allows the energy to flow through more powerfully.

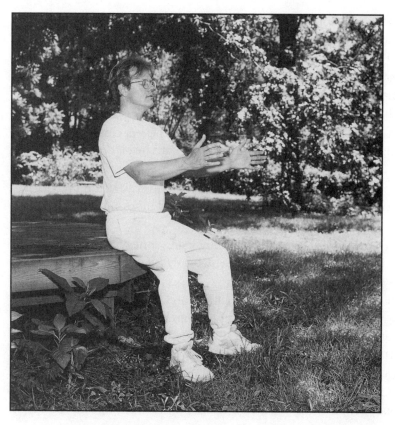

Be sure to let the upper body relax, even though the hands are raised. Slowly move them together and, with eyes closed, open to experience the sensations of Qi in your hands.

32. Slowly, begin to move the palms of your hands toward one another, opening them to the experience of the energy you've begun to gather, not only within and around you but between your palms as well. Move them toward one another, until they are *almost* touching … *and experience*.

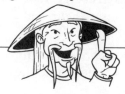

Sage Sifu Says

After learning and regularly practicing the soothing exercise of Sitting QiGong, you will become very adept at it. So, when waiting in line at the supermarket, rather than being bored or anxious, just pretend to be staring at the latest tabloid scandal and open yourself to a soothing flow of life energy as it fills and permeates all the areas where your body is holding onto tension.

33. Good, now slowly move your hands apart until they are about three or four feet away from one another, feeling the difference as they move apart. (Repeat moving hands in and out two more times.)

34. Now, gently place your palms back down on your thighs. With each releasing breath, let all that go, relaxing a bit more into your chair with each exhale.

35. As we let go of that experience, re-open yourself to the downpouring light washing over and through your head and body. With the feet closed, the body is saturated with light. Allow it to spill over the top of your head, quickly filling the field around you.

36. Soon it will feel as though you are floating within a limitlessly expanding ocean of light. With every exhale, allow yourself to be floating more effortlessly within it. *Sit back and enjoy this feeling.*

37. In doing so, you can begin to feel any remaining loads or heavy energy squeezed within the muscles or other tissues being magnetically lifted up and out of the body in all directions.

38. You can literally begin to feel burdens being lifted up and off of the shoulders, *just by breathing and being willing to let go.* Any worries and concerns are lifted off the temples or brow, again just by being willing to let go, and then observing the release. The deep facial muscles release tensions they've held onto during the day.

39. Now any heaviness or angst around the heart begins to be lifted up and off your chest. As the body continues to release these loads, you become aware of your entire being filling with a limitless permeable lightness, refreshing and absolutely effortless.

40. This process of release, cleansing, expanding, and enlightening will continue throughout the day. Even when you're not consciously aware of it, the rhythm of breathing and the willingness to let go will allow you to be lifted into the lightness of this ocean of silken energy. Here your stresses and loads can continually be released into the cleansing light, and your cells and surrounding field will be bathed in its effortless healing.

41. Let yourself sit within this ocean of light, assimilating and soaking in the light. Let go. There is no need to hold onto the light, for *the more we let go, the more there is.*

42. After assimilating the light for a few minutes, very slowly and very gently, when you're ready . . . open your eyes.

The Least You Need to Know

➤ Qi is scientifically observable and measurable.

➤ QiGong is effortless.

➤ Practice Sitting QiGong everyday to supercharge your strength, calm your attitude, and improve your health.

➤ QiGong is a way to program each cell to let go of stress at the earliest indication of blockage.

➤ QiGong programs the mind and body to radiate health.

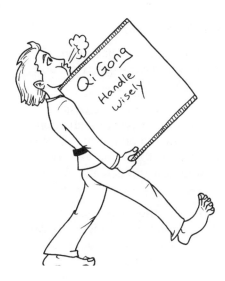

Chapter 12

Moving QiGong (Dong Gong)

In This Chapter

➤ Bone Marrow Cleansing and immune system boost

➤ Moving QiGong cleanses the mind of tension

➤ QiGong promotes elegance

Even walking can be a meditation

➤ QiGong can tonify kidney function

The Sitting QiGong presented in Chapter 11 is a prerequisite for the simple, yet power-ful, Moving QiGong exercises in this chapter. Remember, "mindfulness" is the act of observing, experiencing, and perhaps enjoying, rather than analyzing the world around us *or within us*. Sitting QiGong's effortless mindfulness of truly experiencing yourself from the inside is a big part of how Moving QiGong works its magic.

Here you will experience how Moving QiGong can help treat illnesses and organs. QiGong can enhance immune system responses by cleansing the bone marrow of stress.

The following Moving QiGong exercises will promote elegance and grace in your movements, while also promoting a calm and peaceful state of mind.

Mindful Movement vs. Mindless Exercise

Like Sitting QiGong, the goal of Moving QiGong is to let the mind initiate physical, mental, and emotional releases throughout the body. The more we let go, relax, and open, the more easily and healthfully the energy flows through us.

Much exercise is not very thoughtful. We strain and pound our joints and tissue running on pavement or in other high-impact exercises without paying much attention to the toll it can take on our body. Or for that matter the toll on our mind, as we often listen to loud music or watch the news while scurrying through our exercises. Studies have shown that loud noises and excessive TV watching can actually elevate damaging stress responses.

Moving QiGong, like T'ai Chi, is different. When you practice these exercises, let yourself take a break from the rat race, the noise, and the endless demands of the day. Practice QiGong in silence, hearing only your breath and the motion of your body. Let your mind be filled with the experience of letting go *of everything*.

Bone Marrow Cleansing

Some Moving QiGong exercises have a specific purpose, such as the Bone Marrow Cleansing. As you go through these gentle motions, the energy is encouraged and allowed to flow through the body, even the bone marrow, to cleanse this tissue of frantic energy. The tissue can function at a higher, clearer level if not burdened by old stress.

Hands at chest in prayer position.

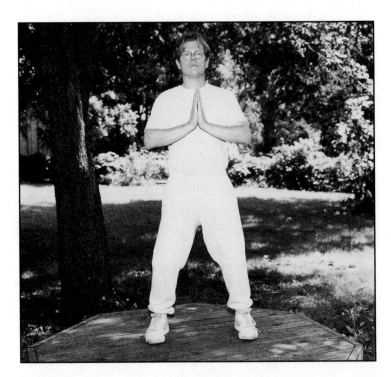

Following are instructions for a Bone Marrow Cleansing QiGong exercise. These will be broken into sections associated with the photographs in this section. The following two instructions will help you practice the movement presented in the previous figure:

1. Bone Marrow Cleansing begins with the feet about shoulder width apart and the knees slightly bent. Your hands are relaxed at your sides.

2. Bring your hands up in front as if lifting a one-foot ball to chest level, then letting the hands come together at the sternum. *Hands at chest in a prayer Position*

Arms out to sides, palms turned outward to universe.

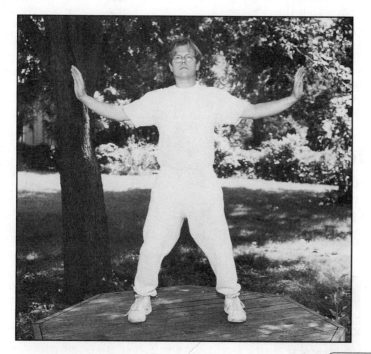

The following two instructions are step-by-step supplements to the figure above:

1. Lower your hands now back down to your sides, and then slowly raise your arms out to the sides.

2. Turn the palms outward. Think of opening the body to absorb the energy of life from the universe. Allow the body and mind to become open and porous.

arms out to sides

T'ai Sci

Many centuries ago before modern microscopes, Chinese health professionals understood that blood and bone marrow were associated with the immune system. They studied exercises like Bone Marrow Cleansing, not by viewing another's cells with a microscope, but by practicing the exercise and then viewing their own internal health responses.

One hand overhead with palm down, and the other hand with back of hand on small of back.

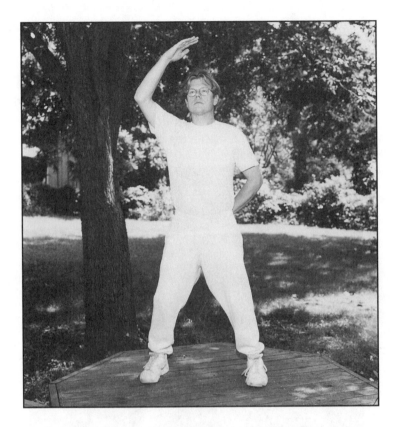

The following four instructions will guide you through the movement depicted in the figure above:

1. Allow your arms to slowly descend to your sides.

2. One hand now floats up and outward away from the body until eventually it is above your head, with the palm turned down toward the top of your head. Meanwhile, the other hand drifts to settle the back of the hand on the small of your back.

3. As the palm above your head turns palm down, allow the energy to pour over and through the head and body. As the hand descends down in front of the body, the body fills with energy, washing through the bones and bone marrow, cleansing the body of any toxins, which are carried right down into the earth through the feet.

4. Repeat this on the other side, each hand now doing what the other did before. Repeat on both sides three times.

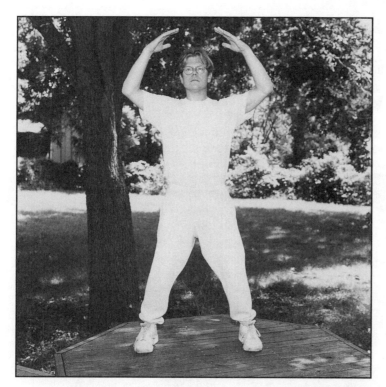

Palms above forehead down, similar to grand terminus.

The following three instructions, with the figure above, guide you through the last section of the Bone Marrow Cleansing exercise:

1. With both arms relaxed at your sides, begin lifting both palms up toward the sky.

2. Push your hands up toward the sky above your head, then turn the palms over facing downward.

3. As the palms float down in front of the body, let the energy pour through the bones and other tissues, carrying any impurities or dense energy right out through the feet into the earth.

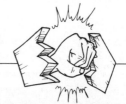

A T'ai Chi Punch Line

Sometimes in classes, students express their concern for the environmental repercussions of releasing their heavy or toxic energy down into the earth. Look at this like our physical human waste, which becomes fodder or nutrients to the earth. Heavy energy the body releases is transmuted and lifted back into a healing force, just like trees breathe our carbon dioxide to create new oxygen. All things balance.

Becoming Elegant with Mulan Quan

Mulan Quan warm ups incorporate several lovely moving QiGong exercises. These promote elegance in movement and carriage, but also have healing effects as well.

Spread Wings to Fly

Spread Wings to Fly is a Moving QiGong exercise that specifically helps with upper limb disorders and to loosen tightness in the shoulders. This is a wonderful exercise to perform during breaks at work to release job tension.

Hands out in front of chest.

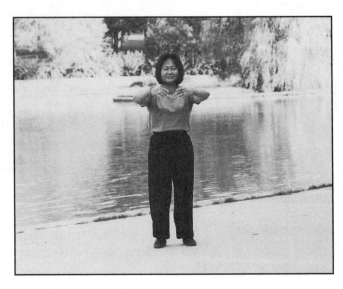

Following are instructions for Spread Wings to Fly:

1. Begin with your hands out in front of your chest (see the figure above). Relax your shoulders and breathe naturally with the tip of the tongue lightly touching the roof of your mouth.

Following are instructions to complete Spread Wings to Fly as seen in the next figure:

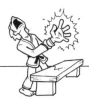

Ouch!

Although all Moving QiGong is likely an excellent addition to any physical therapy you may be involved in, you should use common sense and not force yourself into positions that you are not ready for. Always consult your physician or physical therapist before beginning any new exercise program.

2. Begin a long slow inhalation of breath as you gently pull your arms back around to your sides, until the shoulder blades touch in back, while simultaneously turning your head slowly to the left.

3. Begin exhaling as your arms slowly circle back down and around (rolling out the shoulder sockets) to the start position in front of your chest, while turning your head back to the front.

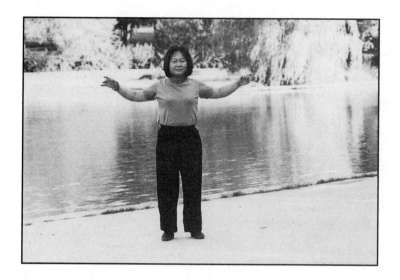

Arms back till shoulder blades touch.

4. Repeat the entire process with your head turning to the right this time.
5. Repeat the process alternately turning your head to the left and then the right, until completing eight forms (four with the head turning to the right, and four with the head turning to the left).

Tupu Spinning

Tupu can be therapeutic for movement limitations of the back, buttocks, legs, knees, and ankles.

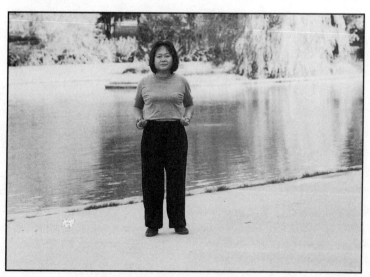

Form fists held at the waist with elbows tucked in and knees slighty bent.

Following is a step-by-step instruction for the previous figure:

1. Begin by forming fists held at the waist, with your elbows tucked in and your knees slightly bent. Breathe normally and easily, yet fully.

Look left, extend right arm out, left shoulder pulling back.

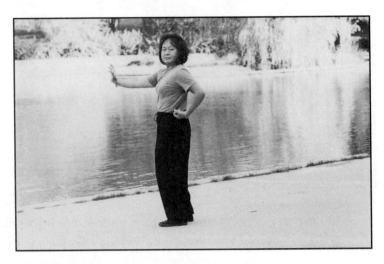

Below are instructions pertaining to the figure above:

2. Inhale as you extend the right shoulder forward and as your right hand pushes out in front of your body. Simultaneously the left shoulder and elbow pull back as you turn your face to look back over your left shoulder. Exhale as you reverse this, pulling your right hand back to square off your shoulders, thereby returning to the start position.

3. Switch, extending your left shoulder out as your left hand pushes, and your right shoulder pulls back as you look back over your right shoulder.

4. Repeat on both sides four times each.

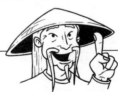

Sage Sifu Says

It is very difficult to fully comprehend how to perform QiGong by reading it from a book. If live classes are unavailable to you, there are many fine QiGong videos available. The Mulan Quan QiGong described in this section is available on the *Mulan Quan Basic Short Form* video listed in the back of this book.

Bring Knee to Chest

This movement not only feels great, but it also helps with any pain in the legs and buttocks and is therapy for functional disorders of the leg involving bending and extending.

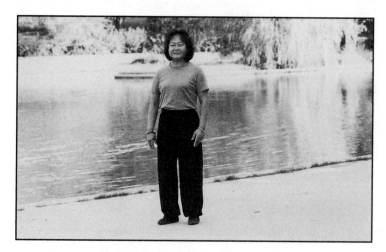

Hands at sides relaxed, knees bent.

The instruction below is for the figure above:

1. Begin with your hands relaxed at your sides, your knees slightly bent, while breathing easily and naturally.

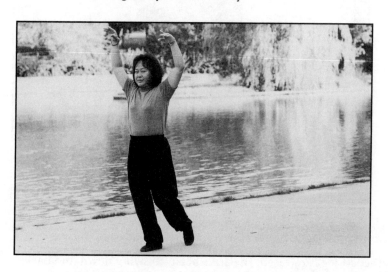

Step forward with right leg, swing arms backward.

Refer to the following instructions for the figure above:

2. Now begin inhaling as you step forward with your right leg, shifting your weight to the right leg as your arms swing upward and back in great round arcs.

3. As the arms' arcs begin to swing down and toward the front, the left leg begins to lift.

Lift left knee, wrap hands around knee.

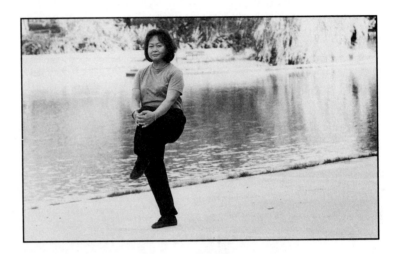

The following instruction is for the figure above:

4. Lift up your left knee in front, pointing the toes of the left foot down, and wrap your hands around your knee to help it stretch up gently.

Left leg steps back behind as arms swing up and over.

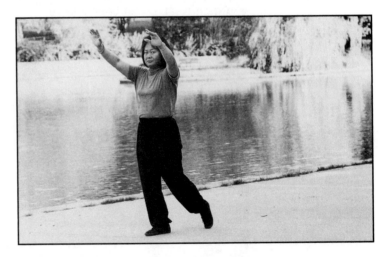

The following instructions are for the figure above:

5. Now exhale. As the left leg is released, the arms begin to swing down and back.

6. Place your left foot behind you and shift the weight back onto the left leg as your arms swing from the back over the top toward the front.

7. Allow the right leg to come back even with the left, as your hands descend, returning you to the start position.

8. Repeat with the left leg stepping out this time. Repeat the entire process alternating sides (four times on each side).

Zen Walking in the Old Soft Shoe

Zen meditations involve a mindfulness that simultaneously allows your mind let go of the worries of the world, while attuning yourself to the world in a clear and healing way. Zen walking is a common T'ai Chi exercise. It teaches us how to let our movement fill our mind, while improving our balance and dexterity.

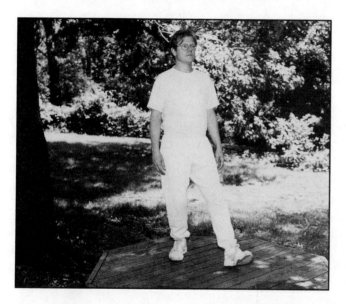

Zen walking resembles the way Groucho Marx used to walk.

Place the heel of one foot outward at a slight angle, while maintaining balance over the back foot. Remember to breathe easily and naturally when Zen walking.

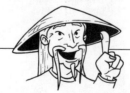

Sage Sifu Says

Just as Zen walking makes a meditation or relaxation therapy out of simple walking, we can expand this ability throughout our lives. T'ai Chi and QiGong's teaching of mindful awareness of the subtleties of life can help us make anything we do a meditation, whether it's washing dishes or paying bills. In doing so, every moment becomes more healthful, pleasant, and meaningful.

157

Ouch!

Although QiGong may help with premature hair loss, it works best as part of an overall healthful lifestyle. So, if you are in a high-pressure job you hate, aren't getting enough sleep, and smoking too much, the benefits of QiGong will be limited. QiGong practice may help you sleep better and eventually quit smoking. Therefore, QiGong should be viewed not as a cure-all, but as a stairway to a healthier lifestyle.

Assume the position in the previous figure, and then follow the instructions below:

1. Slowly shift your dan tien, or weight, up toward the front foot, while slowly rolling the foot down onto the ground.

2. The back foot stays flat until your vertical axis, or dan tien, is settled over the front foot. Now let your heel lift up, then the foot, and now bring that foot up near your weight bearing foot, before placing it out in front at a slight angle just like in the beginning.

3. This can be repeated many times, all the way across your living room or backyard. The goal is to do it enough so that you forget about everything in the world except the soles of your feet, the ground they contact, and the shifting tissue in your body.

Carry the Moon

As discussed in Chapter 3, QiGong can treat specific organs, or systems, in the body. Carry the Moon is great for keeping the spine supple and can also tonify kidney function. It has been said that this may also help reduce premature baldness. This may be because, as with all QiGong and T'ai Chi, it promotes circulation, but in the case of Carry the Moon, especially in the scalp.

Leaning over with hands hanging down to about knees.

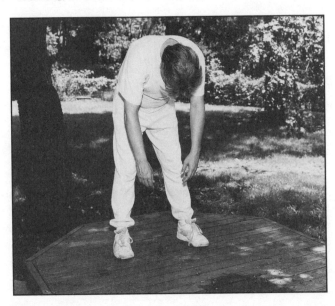

Carry the Moon begins with letting your hands and head simply hang loosely over as you bend effortlessly forward. Do not try to strain, as if attempting to touch your toes. Just let yourself hang comfortably, with your hands at about knee level or higher.

Breathe naturally and easily.

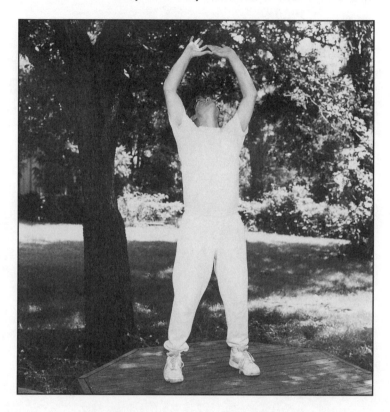

With hands above head forming a circle between thumb and forefingers, looking through it.

Use the following instructions in conjunction with the figure above:

1. Form a circle using the thumbs and forefingers of both hands. As you slowly rise up the hands ascend up above your head.

2. Let the hands go up and slightly back behind as you gently arch your back to look up through the circle your hands form.

3. Hold this position as you breathe effortlessly and naturally for a few moments, then let yourself hang forward again, and begin again. Repeat several times.

The Least You Need to Know

➤ Sitting QiGong prepared you for moving QiGong.

➤ Breath and mindfulness is important in QiGong.

➤ QiGong can improve all organ functions.

➤ QiGong may slow premature hair loss.

➤ Use QiGong as a launch pad to a healthier you.

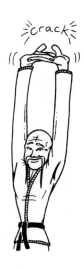

Warm Ups

T'ai Chi warm-up exercises are not only meant to warm the muscle and other tissues but also to center the mind as well. You cannot listen to the radio or watch TV while warming up for T'ai Chi.

Unlike the way many of us were taught to "stretch" out our muscles when warming up by using straining stances, T'ai Chi warm ups start from the very center of our being. We begin by becoming self-aware of that center and then relaxing ourselves from the deep skeletal muscles outward. We prepare ourselves for fluid and effortless movement by allowing our body to relax around our breathing lungs, and then all the muscles relax on top of the moving skeleton.

Each warm up is a form of QiGong and promotes health and healing on many levels. These warm ups are a beneficial exercise program even without T'ai Chi, but T'ai Chi offers so much more.

Dan Tien Takes Us for a Ride

When we start our Sitting QiGong, warm ups, or T'ai Chi movements, our mind is usually scattered. We are thinking about what we need to do at work, what we need to do to prepare dinner tonight, and so on. So the first task of warm ups is to center our mind, and the center of our being is as you know, the dan tien.

Breathing Our Way to Center

There is nothing more calming and centering than hearing and feeling your own breath. Therefore all T'ai Chi–related exercises begin by simply closing your eyes and feeling the rhythm of your own breathing. The following points explain this in detail:

➤ Let your eyes close easily and naturally as you stand comfortably with feet fairly close together and knees slightly bent.

➤ Notice how your lungs fill and empty. Think of breathing into the bottom or abdominal part of the lungs, then letting the top or chest area fill.

➤ As you breathe, allow the muscles in your head and torso to let go. This allows the breaths to become not only deeper but also more and more effortless, almost as if the breath were beginning to breathe you.

➤ Let your awareness or mind relax, riding on the rhythm of your own breath.

➤ Now, think of breathing down into the dan tien area. You can experience the slight expanse of the upper pelvic muscles as you breath in, and how those muscles relax in as you release the breath.

➤ You may experience a feeling of air expanding down into that area. Of course the lungs don't go down that far, so you are feeling the Qi, or your awareness, expanding through the dan tien area.

Let the Dan Tien Do the Driving

The breathing exercises help your awareness expand in the dan tien area, which prepares you to let the dan tien be the movement. This may sound a little odd at first, but after playing the following exercises for a while, it'll be quite natural and will dramatically improve your focus, balance, and movement. The first two T'ai Chi warm-up exercises help you to practice this and are explained in the following figures.

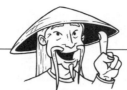

Sage Sifu Says

If you are in a wheelchair or have an injury or condition that requires you to sit, let the most inner part of your upper pelvis go into motion and be aware of that motion, allowing the body to relax as much as possible around that motion. If you are paralyzed, let the internal rotation begin in the center of the body at the lowest point your physical awareness begins.

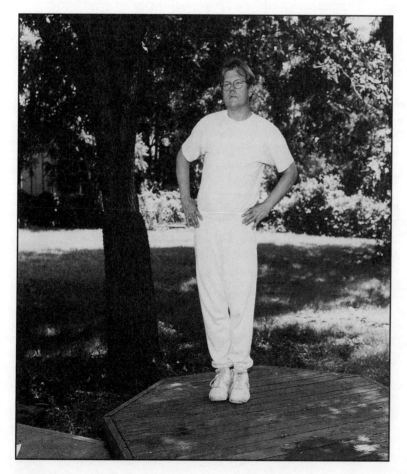

Feet together rotating hips in hula hoop fashion.

With your feet close together, let the dan tien, or hips, begin a counterclockwise rotation, sort of like a hula hoop motion. If you were looking down at a clock face beneath your feet, you would be going counterclockwise. Notice that the dan tien begins to move effortlessly like a gyroscope in motion, allowing you to let your muscles relax while the dan tien moves the skeleton underneath. The shoulders do not move too much; most of the motion is in the dan tien, or hip area. However, don't be rigid about this. The goal is to get loose.

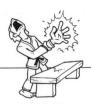

Ouch

If your balance is too unstable on the first set of rotations with feet close together and eyes closed, open your eyes, but soften your focus so that your awareness can still go inside. You will find that when you move to the second exercise of rotations with the feet shoulder width apart, your balance will be more secure.

Repeat the counterclockwise hip rotations 32 times, if that feels good to you, and then repeat 32 in the opposite direction, clockwise.

Close your eyes as you rotate the dan tien. At first this may challenge your balance, but you'll get better. With eyes closed your awareness can go within. You will notice areas of the body loosening as you rotate and breathe. Think of letting the muscles let go of bones and other tissue, allowing the body to just generally loosen on top of the skeleton. You will notice the lower back vertebrae loosening as the muscles around them begin to let go. You will also notice this loosening spreading up the back through the lumbar region, up through the dorsal vertebrae between the shoulders, and into the neck and back of the head. Basically, anywhere you let your light of awareness shine within, your body, mind, or heart can begin to loosen as you breathe effortlessly and move effortlessly in these dan tien rotations.

Now, repeat the hip rotations both ways (first counterclockwise and then clockwise), with your feet about shoulder width apart, and again knees slightly bent. Relax and enjoy the sensations of movement. With the feet farther apart and eyes closed, you will notice that you can very tangibly feel the top of the femur or hipbone rotating in the hip socket. Slow the rotations down, and you will feel the hipbone rotating all the way around the inner rim of the hip socket.

Enjoy the deep-tissue massage that the rotating bones give, as the deep hip muscles begin to let go of the tensions built up there. As you breathe and let muscles relax on top of the moving skeleton, you can enjoy this loosening through the back, legs, and rest of the body.

The enjoyment of this internal loosening helps us almost "see inside ourselves." Practicing this pleasant internal vision is a powerful health tool. By becoming aware of how good effortless motion feels inside, we also become aware of tensions or "diseases" at a very early stage before they actually become diseases.

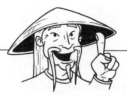

Sage Sifu Says

We are a very shallow-breathing society. Therefore, you may catch yourself breathing very shallowly or even holding your breath as you move. Let your lungs fill effortlessly all the way down to the abdominal region and up to the top. Allow the entire body to relax that breath out, as if every cell of the body were letting go at the deepest level with each breath. Each breath lets us practice living effortlessly. There is nothing more effortless than the release of a breath.

Lengthened, Not Stretched

In T'ai Chi warm ups, we don't strain to stretch out muscles. We allow ourselves to "lengthen" until we begin to ease up against strain. The tension we become aware of indicates a block. Then, we take a deep breath, and as we exhale, we allow light, or Qi, to fill the area of tension or restriction, which lets the block begin to let go. You can actually feel the lightness or release spread effortlessly through a tight or restraining muscle as you let the breath out. The mind's awareness of the block directs the Qi, or energy, into the center of the block as you let the breath relax out of the body.

Fingers interlaced stretching upward.

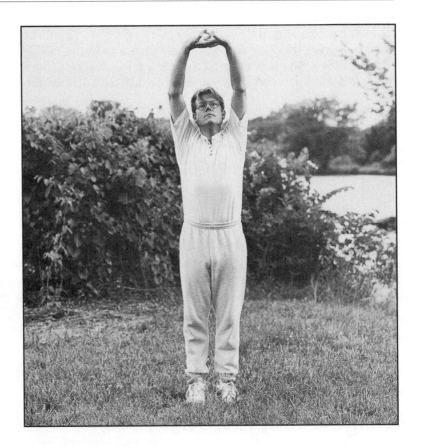

1. With fingers interlaced, extend your hands up over your head.

2. Don't stretch, but allow your body to be effortlessly lengthened, as if the hands were being lifted up toward the sky.

3. As you release each sighing exhale, think of letting the muscles beneath the muscles let go.

4. Enjoy the feeling of effortless release through the back, shoulders, neck, head, and down into the hips and legs. As we breathe and let go, the entire body gets a bit of a stretch.

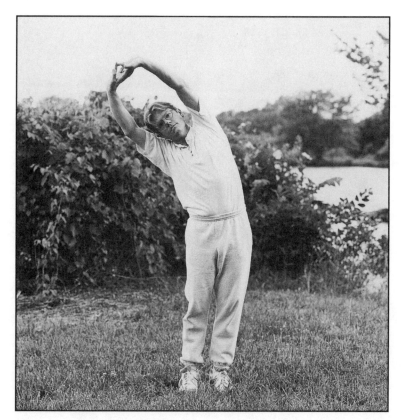

Hands extended but now stretching over sideways.

Along with the figure above, the following instructions will guide you through this exercise:

1. Now stretch out to either side, but rather than thinking of stretching, think of the hands being drawn out and upward toward the sky out to the left and then the right. First the hands are drawn outward and up off to the right side of the body, and then easing back upward and over to the left side.

2. Go back and forth. Do not stretch so far to the side that it is a big strain. Rather, go just far enough that you can savor the sensation of the muscles stretching across the back, between the shoulders and through the neck. Again, as we loosen, the entire body gets a bit of a soothing effortless stretch.

Back bent flat, with hands hanging down.

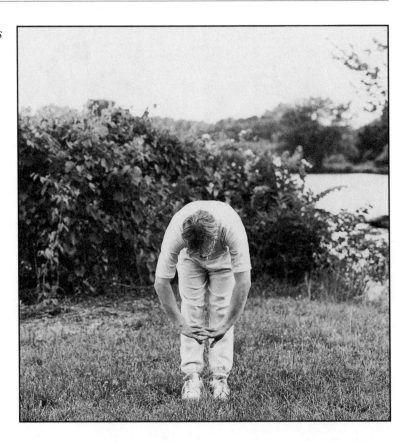

Using the figure above and the following instructions, relax into this effortless posture.

1. Now, lengthen straight up again before stretching out and forward. The back should be fairly straight, bending from the hips and letting the arms just hang down.

2. Do not strain to touch your toes. That's not the point. The point is to feel an effortless lengthening through the upper body as we simply let go.

3. Enjoy that feeling of effortless elongation through the shoulders, neck, and back of the head. Notice that with each releasing exhale you can let go even more. With each releasing breath the muscles in the head can let go even more, showing you that relaxation is not a destination, but an endlessly enriching process of letting go.

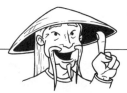

Sage Sifu Says

When doing all T'ai Chi warm-up exercises, let your eyes close so that your awareness can relax within. Enjoy the sensations of loosening and breath. Breathe fully, but don't force yourself. Breathe easily and naturally.

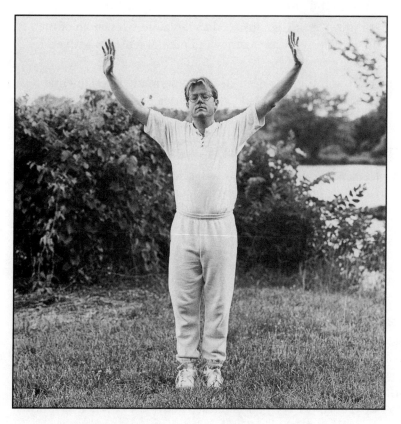

Hands descending to the sides.

Use the figure above and the following instructions to deeply let go.

1. Slowly and gently straighten back up to the original position of the figure above, with hands high over the head interlaced.

169

2. With eyes closed, take a deep breath and on the sighing exhale, allow the hands to descend to the sides so slowly that you can feel the air passing between the fingers. As the hands arc down from above the head out to the sides and the breath relaxes out, experience the different muscle groups letting go through the head, face, jaw, neck, shoulders, torso, arms, legs, and even into the hands and feet.

3. Let each exhale trigger a deep letting go from the very center of your being, as if the bones themselves could let go. Let every cell in the body relax those breaths out.

4. As you stand with your eyes closed, let go of all the muscles with each breath, and also let go of the heart. Just as the muscles release tensions with each sigh or yawn, the heart can let go of tensions or loads that it has squeezed in the heart muscle or muscles around the heart.

5. Think of the brain or mind letting go. Just as the cranial muscles let go of their grip on the skull, the mind can release worries and mental tensions with each releasing breath.

6. Realize that each breath can trigger a deep cleansing on many levels, mental, emotional, and physical. With each exhale, experience a deep letting go.

Filling the Sandbags, Sinking the Qi

Settling down into the Horse Stance is sinking our weight down into both feet as if we were sinking down into a saddle on a horse. Again, the tailbone drops as the pelvis tilts slightly up, and the head is drawn upward toward the sky, while the chin is pulled slightly in. This causes the spine to lengthen, which is great for the back, releasing a lot of the pressure daily stress puts on it.

Moving from the Horse Stance not only improves posture and balance, but it can also preserve our joints and make us more powerful.

Moving from the Horse Stance

Once you settle in the Horse Stance, let the dan tien flow back and forth from one leg to the other. Picture yourself sitting on an office chair with wheels, rolling from side to side. Or as if you were sitting on the back of a park bench, sliding your bottom from side to side. Notice that the head and shoulder never lead the way, nor do the hips stick out from side to side. The upper body stays stacked above the dan tien as it flows back and forth.

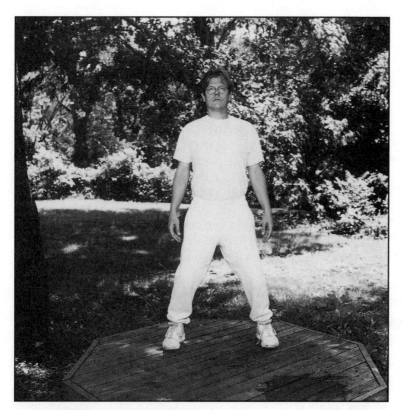

Note that the knees in the Horse Stance are slightly bent, and the upper body is stacked above the dan tien, erect but relaxed and not rigid.

As you become aware of discomfort or tension—the fatigue you may feel in the muscles above the knees, for example—play the following game.

1. Let yourself feel the tension or discomfort, wherever it is in your body.
2. Experience how it feels and where you feel it.
3. Now, as you let the next breath out, think of letting the light, or Qi, expand right in the center of that feeling.
4. Let your awareness sit back and enjoy whatever responses you experience. Often you will experience a lessening of the discomfort or even a pleasure of the expanding lightness.

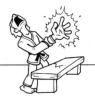

Ouch

Do not feel as though you must do all T'ai Chi exercises, such as the Deep Sinking Qi exercise. Whatever warm ups fit your abilities are the ones you should do. However, you may be able to modify exercises to fit your ability. If you are in a wheelchair or must sit while performing T'ai Chi, develop upper body stretches you can perform while the rest of the class is doing leg stretches.

Sinking the Qi

In T'ai Chi, the upper body does not lean but stays stacked up above the dan tien, just like in the Horse Stance. The dan tien flowing toward one leg fills that leg with the Qi, or energy (or the weight of your body). Simultaneously, the leg that the dan tien moves away from is emptying of Qi, or weight. In T'ai Chi, we rarely ever pivot a leg that has weight on it because it makes your balance precarious. More importantly, it damages the knees to pivot feet that bear weight. So, this Moving from the Dan Tien exercise teaches us to shift our weight from one leg to the other. This simple exercise is the most important T'ai Chi warm up because this is what T'ai Chi is. All of T'ai Chi's elaborate forms are based on the dan tien moving from one leg to another.

Flowing upper body to the other side.

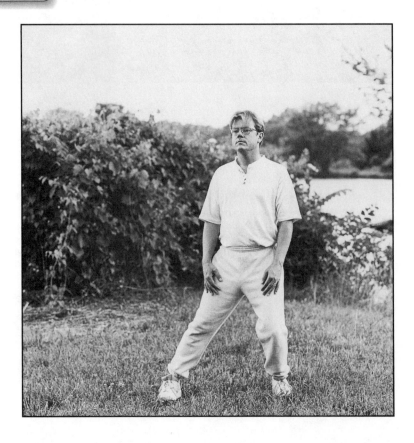

172

Adventurously Sinking Your Qi

If your mobility permits and you feel adventurous, you can practice a deep sinking of the Qi exercise, illustrated in the following figure.

Note that as the dan tien drops deeply down into one leg by bending that knee, the back is not bent over. As always, we do not bend, keeping the upper body stacked up above the dan tien.

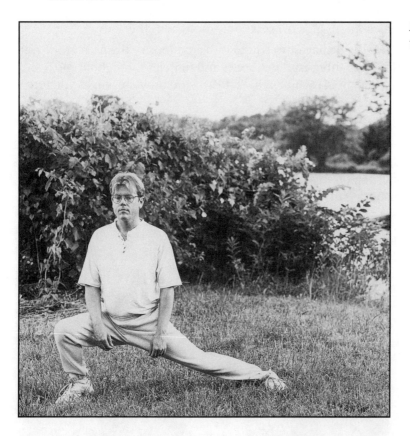

Deep bending of one knee with back straight.

The Chinese Drum's Kaleidoscopic Sensations

The Chinese Drum mimics the motion of those little toy drums with the two swinging beads. When the drum is turned from side to side the beads twist and drum alternately on each side. This is how your relaxed arms and hands will gently strike your body, as you follow the instructions below and refer to the next two figures.

1. Now stand up with feet about shoulder width apart and knees, as always, slightly bent. Gently turn swinging arms out. The lead arm swings across the back to strike the flank or lower back, as the trailing arm swings across the front of the body to strike the shoulder.

2. As the hands strike the shoulder and flank in back, close your eyes and enjoy the physical contact. The gentle slapping begins to massage the muscles, as you turn back and forth, alternately slapping each flank and shoulder in turn.

3. Let your mind release any analytical or problem-solving thoughts and simply open to the pleasure of the motion.

4. With each turn and releasing breath, allow the body to let go even more.

5. Let the mind relax into the pleasure of that letting go, allowing the mind to experience the tens of thousands of sensations throughout the body.

6. With eyes closed, we can attune ourselves to the sensations of the pads of the feet shifting on the floor, the interactions of bones and muscles throughout the body, and the releasing pleasure of each breath. Feel the wind on your skin as you turn through space.

7. Even with closed eyes, patterns of light and shadow flow across your eyelids, and sounds both internal and external flow over and through you.

8. Do not try to hear, feel, or see. Rather, let your mind relax and allow sensations, images, and sounds to pour over and through your mind the way clear mountain water pours over a waterfall.

Turning and arm swinging out from body.

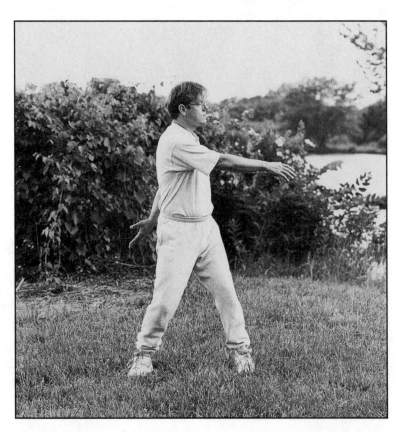

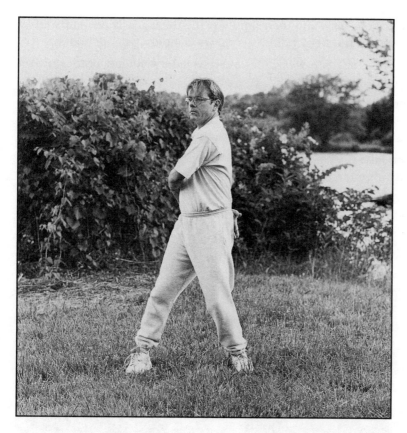

Hands striking body in back and shoulder.

Let the mind give up straining to function or reaching out to the world, but rather allow the world to flow to you in a soothing experience of effortlessness. Think of your mind releasing its grip on the dock of logical thought and floating down a river of kaleidoscopic sensation, carried on the beauty of existence, savoring the ability to breathe, flow, and experience sensation . . . effortlessly.

Deep-Tissue Cleansing Leaves You Radiant

QiGong provides many deep-tissue cleansing exercises, and the following is only one. It contains two parts that should be practiced gently and, as always, with awareness of your own mobility range.

Flinging Off and Breathing Out Toxins

Most tensions that we carry around are energy we've squeezed in our mind, heart, and the muscles in the body. You know this is true because on days when you feel heavy and weighted down by the world, if you get on a scale you don't weigh any more than usual. Therefore, we can simply fling off much of the loads we lug around.

1. Begin with hands above head and then simply swing them gently outward and downward, flinging off the weight of the world we've holding in our bodies.

2. Think of letting the bone marrow itself release the load it's holding onto, which of course it can release.

3. As the hands fling toward the ground, think of the hands and feet opening to release that load to fly out of us into the cleansing earth. As your hands swing out and down, exhale deeply to facilitate the release.

4. Breathe in as you raise the hands back up over the head, and again release all as you swing the hands out and down again. Repeat several times.

Hands up high ready to swing out and down.

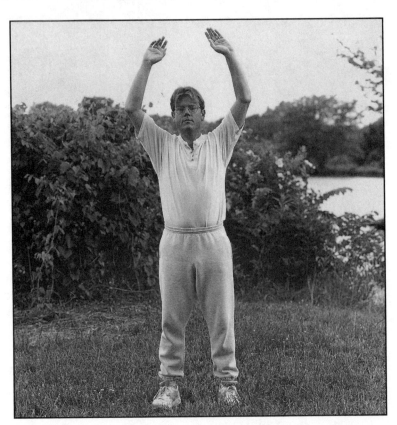

Elvis Impersonations Cleanse the Soul—Baby!

This tissue-cleansing exercise looks very much like an Elvis impersonation. With feet about shoulder width apart, eyes closed, and knees slightly bent, just shake. Gently let the arms and entire body go liquid and shake. Do not jolt the joints, but allow a liquid rippling to wave through every muscle and joint. Experience the skeletal muscles jiggling on the bones, from the top of the head to the pads of the feet. It's very slight and very subtle, but as those muscles loosen, they begin to cleanse the body of deep toxins. Think of the brain and heart loosening as well, letting worries, angst, and tensions evaporate out of the body with each yawn or sighing exhale.

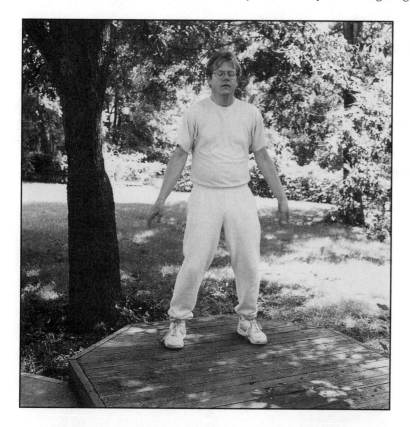

Let yourself go as liquid and limp as you can, with eyes closed enjoying a loosening throughout your being.

Have one last good series of shakes while taking in a nice full breath. On the long sighing exhale, stop shaking and just feel the body awakening. Notice how every cell fills with an effortless lightness, clear, clean, and alive. Wherever you notice remaining tension or block, with each releasing breath allow the light to expand with that area as if the body were expanding endlessly outward, releasing any heavy loads to evaporate in that endless lighted expansion.

T'ai Sci

There are blood lactates, or lactic acids, which accumulate in the deep skeletal muscles during times of anxiety. Studies also show that these acids produce anxiety. Therefore, T'ai Chi and warm ups like the Elvis Impersonation or Tissue Cleansing allow the body to release these long-held anxieties and to cleanse itself of them.

177

The Least You Need to Know

➤ The dan tien makes all movement effortless.

➤ Let warm ups loosen your entire being.

➤ Moving from the Horse Stance is the most important warm-up exercise.

➤ The Chinese Drum cleans your mind and body.

➤ Let the exercises be a sensory amusement park.

➤ Doing warm ups with eyes closed helps the mind relax within.

Part 4

Kuang Ping T'ai Chi: Walk on Life's Lighter Side

Part 4 is an introduction to the Kuang Ping Yang Right Style's 20-minute long form. Chapter 14 will prepare you mentally for the physical experience presented in the following chapters. You will learn how T'ai Chi movements aid certain organs, and what T'ai Chi has in common with the ancient Chinese I-Ching, or The Book of Changes. The remaining chapters in Part 4 illustrate the 64 postures of Kuang Ping Yang style's forms, and text will explain some of the transition movements that link them together. Many of these forms can be seen performed in other styles of T'ai Chi as well. So the explanations of the benefits each movement provides and the T'ai Chi principles explained can also benefit those practicing other forms.

Yet no matter how you learn your forms, once your entire 20-minute form is learned, it becomes a gateway to another state of mind. The constant effortless focus on the pleasure of movement and relaxed breathing, coupled with the concentration demanded by gravity and balance, brings your mind, heart, and body to a place of tranquil calm. As you learn and practice T'ai Chi, you will constantly ask yourself one recurring question, "How did I ever get along without this?"

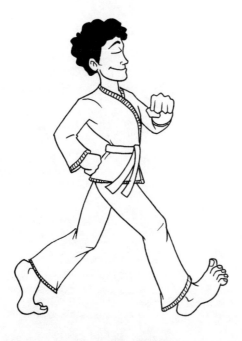

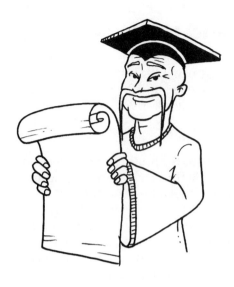

Chapter 14

Kuang Ping Yang Style History

In This Chapter

➤ T'ai Chi's ancient roots

➤ How T'ai Chi became a philosophy of life

➤ How T'ai Chi makes us feel connected

➤ Long forms versus short forms

➤ Historical roots of medicine and T'ai Chi intertwine

This style of T'ai Chi has a rich and colorful history, as do all the ancient styles. The history of T'ai Chi is a great way to better understand its benefits and why it is so perfect for our modern harried lives.

This chapter will discuss the roots of all T'ai Chi and explain how Kuang Ping Yang and the more extant Yang style became different. You will also learn why some styles offer shortened versions and why Kuang Ping has not developed a short form.

Understanding some of the historical or ancient tenets of T'ai Chi may actually help you get many more and endlessly richer benefits from its practice. The more your mind believes in your therapy, the more powerfully it heals.

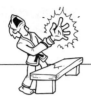

Ouch!

If the idea of learning a long T'ai Chi form that may take 8 to 12 months to learn is daunting, remember the following: The journey of a thousand miles begins under one's own feet.

The Snake and the Hawk

According to legend, T'ai Chi was born from an observation of nature. A martial arts master observed how a snake slowly evaded a crane's attack by moving away each time the crane's sharp beak struck. What may have been mortal combat became a gentle exercise that left the exhausted crane flying off for easier prey.

This example of yielding to the brute force of the world has created not only a powerful martial art but also an extremely healthful philosophy for surviving the stressful onslaught of an accelerating future. If this crane's attacks are compared with today's rapid changes, we may be much smarter to bend and yield to that change than to dig our heels in and fight it. The snake's yielding was much less stressful than a head to head fight with the larger, sharp-beaked crane.

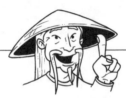

Sage Sifu Says

Master Henry Look, one of the original students of Master Kuo Lien Ying of China, says there are seven important principles to T'ai Chi.

➤ Centering   ➤ Quiet movement

➤ Focus   ➤ Quiet breathing

➤ Coordination   ➤ Quiet smile

➤ Quiet mind

The Shao-Lin Temple: Where It All Began

The Shao-Lin Temple that was featured on the famous television series *Kung Fu* is actually where T'ai Chi began. An 18-movement stretching exercise that eventually grew into T'ai Chi was taught to the monks by a man known as Ta Mo around 400 AD. The purported founder of modern T'ai Chi, however, was a monk named Chang San-feng, who lived about a thousand years later. It was Chang San-feng who is said to have watched the snake yield and avoid the crane's harsh attacks.

From the Temple to the West

The Chen family, founders of the Chen style of T'ai Chi, created one of the earliest family styles. The Chen style was taught to a young martial artist named Yang Lu-chan, who was the founder of today's Yang style.

The Yang family taught a style of T'ai Chi while residing in the city of Kuang Ping. Here the founding master Yang Lu-chan's eldest son, Yang Pan-hou, was made an offer *he couldn't refuse* to teach T'ai Chi at the imperial court and become the emperor's personal teacher. Since Yang could not refuse the emperor, he decided to create a lesser version of the family style to teach him, one that was inferior to the real Kuang Ping Yang Style, which was practical, powerful, and a highly effective self-defense system.

This Kuang Ping Yang style was passed down from Yang Pan-hou to his student Wong Jao-yu, who taught master Kuo Lien Ying who eventually migrated to the United States and taught this to students who have since spread this style all across the U.S.

This can be about as difficult to sort out as the cast of a soap opera, so don't worry about these details. It's just important to remember that the tools you are about to enjoy are the fruits of centuries of study. I include these stories not to confuse but to acknowledge and to thank these people for making available all that T'ai Chi has to offer.

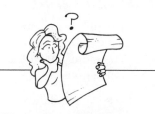

Know Your Chinese

Chinese names begin with the family name. Therefore **Yang Lu-chan**, founder of the Yang style, would be called Lu-chan Yang in the West, as Yang is his family name.

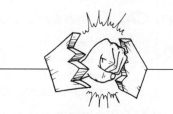

A T'ai Chi Punch Line

T'ai Chi styles have been created with the same fluidity to the world's demands that T'ai Chi encourages its practitioners to have. For example, the Wu style was created by Wu Quan-yu, a palace guard in the Imperial Court who designed a system of T'ai Chi that could be performed in the restrictive clothing of an imperial palace guard's uniform.

T'ai Chi Becomes a Philosophy

Around 1500 AD, the Taoist philosopher Wan Yang-ming began to blend the gentle centering philosophical concepts of Taoism into the equally centering physical concepts of T'ai Chi. This gave practitioners a real way to live a more healing, nonviolent life—not just preaching it or thinking about it, but actually training their mind and body how to live that way through T'ai Chi's gentle mind/body fitness program. The modern styles now widely practiced, Yang, Chen, Wu, Mulan Quan, and others all incorporate the beautiful personal growth concepts of Taoist philosophy.

T'ai Chi Links Man to Nature

The philosophy of T'ai Chi is based on the idea of the balance of nature, both internally in our health systems and externally in our relationships with the natural world. Therefore you will see nature imitated in many of the T'ai Chi form names, such as the following:

➤ Wave Hands Like Clouds

➤ Wind Blowing Lotus Leaves

➤ White Crane Cools Its Wings

➤ Retreat to Ride the Tiger

The poetic quality of these names does more than just remind us how to perform the movements. On a subliminal level, they make us feel more at home in the natural world, somehow more attuned to our connection to the whole of life.

T'ai Chi Connects Us to the Universe

T'ai Chi movement names can also help us remember our multidimensional nature. We are physical and mental beings, of course, and T'ai Chi integrates these aspects of ourselves well, but it connects our minds and bodies with our spirit or energy nature as well. This connection is reflected in movement names, such as:

➤ Strike Palm to Ask Blessing

➤ Focus Mind Towards the Temple

T'ai Chi reminds that we are part of the universe, and that in fact we are made of the same energy that stars and everything else are made of. T'ai Chi is meant to open us up to the limitless supply of energy within us, in the earth we walk upon, and from the universe our world hurtles through. That universal connection is also reflected in movement names:

➤ Step Up to Form Seven Stars

➤ Grand Terminus, the final movement, opens us up to the limitless energy of the universe around us

Advantages of the Long Forms

Today, there are several short versions of the original long forms. Although these shortened versions serve useful purposes, such as enabling a student to acquire a practice system more quickly, there may have been a reason for the average 20-minute length of some of the long forms. The value of a 20-minute-long form is now borne out in modern medical research.

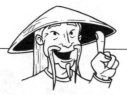

Sage Sifu Says

Most short forms of T'ai Chi take between 8 to 10 minutes. If you practice a short form, simply loop it twice so that you can exercise for 20 minutes and get more benefit. However, if you ever get an opportunity to learn the long form of your style, do it. The complexity of 20 minutes of different movements keeps your mind in a state of relaxed focus, even more so than repetition of the same movements does.

We now know the original ancient forms, which usually took a minimum of 20 minutes to complete, were that length for a good reason. In the ground-breaking book *The Relaxation Response*, by Dr. Herbert Benson, it was noted that a 20-minute relaxation response exercise seemed to evoke the optimum benefits. Apparently, the first few minutes of a relaxation therapy are used by the mind to just wind down; the remaining time truly allows the deep alpha state relaxation these therapies are known for.

It is highly advisable, therefore, to take the time to learn a long form of T'ai Chi.

Why 64 Movements?

While the more extensive Yang form names 108 movements, the Kuang Ping Yang style long form claims 64 movements.

There may be more to this than just chance. The number 64 has profound philosophical meaning. The Chinese classic *I-Ching,* or *The Book of Changes,* is an ancient text of divination and philosophy that attempts to explain how the universal forces of Yin and Yang ebb and flow, combine and disintegrate, and rise and fall to create the dance of existence. The central premise is that all things are in a constant state of change, including our lives and us. T'ai Chi's goal is to help us flow with the change and not be compulsively attached to the old *or the new,* using what works and discarding what is no longer useful. As if you were a surfer riding the changing waves of life, let go of old waves as they recede, to ease onto the mounting power of the new wave.

The *I-Ching* uses Trigrams or figures with three lines (pictured in the following figure to symbolize the changes in life). When two Trigrams are combined, 64 possible combinations are obtained. These 64 hexagrams are said to represent all possible states of change in the universe. Therefore, Kuang Ping Yang's 64 flowing movements symbolize and in some ways physically help us to flow through all the possible changes and challenges of life those changes entail.

Trigrams are combinations of three lines, which can be broken in half or be whole, making eight possible combinations.

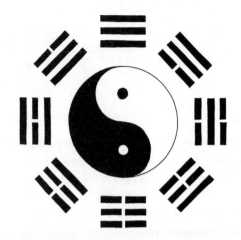

T'ai Sci

Some T'ai Chi movements look very similar to modern physical therapies. For example, Dropping the Duck's Beak, which is an extension of the fingers bending down to touch the thumb, is the same as a Carpal Tunnel prevention exercise used in many corporations. It appears that the therapy for modern repetitive stress disorders may have been discovered centuries ago.

That Kuang Ping Yang style T'ai Chi forms involve 64 movements may have deeper reasons than we know. The complexity and powerful healing qualities that T'ai Chi offers are only now beginning to be discovered by modern science. There may be many other details of how and why T'ai Chi does what it does that will be uncovered in years to come.

T'ai Chi's Movements and Chinese Medicine

As you read in Chapter 3, Traditional Chinese Medicine uses the Zang Fu system of understanding how organs interact. Each of these organ systems is represented by one of the five elements of the Earth, according to ancient Chinese physics.

➤ Metal = Lungs and large intestines

➤ Wood = Liver and gall bladder

➤ Water = Bladder and kidney

➤ Fire = Heart/pericardium/small intestine/triple warmer

➤ Earth = Spleen and stomach

T'ai Chi movements are described with this same system, and the motion of the body that T'ai Chi promotes may have a healing effect on those systems. The directions of movement each correlate to one of the earth elements.

Movement Directions Relative to the Body:

➤ Metal = Advance

➤ Wood = Retreat

➤ Water = Left

➤ Fire = Right

➤ Earth = Center

Movement Directions Relative to Earth:

➤ Metal = West

➤ Wood = East

➤ Water = North

➤ Fire = South

➤ Earth = Center

Ouch!

It is not important to mentally calculate what movement or direction benefits what system of the body. It is more important to simply allow the mind and body to enjoy the exquisite pleasure of effortless breath and movement as you do T'ai Chi. Rest assured that each aspect of your mind, heart, and body is being nourished and healed by the life energy T'ai Chi practice promotes.

The 64 postures of the Kuang Ping Yang style take about 20 minutes to complete. The movements flow in an unending progression from one to the next until the final movement, the Grand Terminus. The movements will move the body outward and backward in all the directions described above. There is also a meditative quality to that motion that cannot be described or conveyed in print.

The following chapters in this section will, however, provide photographs of each of the 64 Kuang Ping Yang style movements, numbered in sequence. They will explain many of the benefits of each movement, pointers on correctly performing them, and cautionary notes to help your T'ai Chi experience be both healthy and profound.

A video will greatly enhance the book's explanations of movements, if live classes are unavailable to you.

The Least You Need to Know

➤ T'ai Chi teaches us to yield when life attacks and advance when opportunities open.

➤ 20-minute-long forms have advantages over short forms.

➤ The 64 Kuang Ping movements ease the mind and body through changes.

➤ T'ai Chi movements have healing abilities we've yet to completely understand.

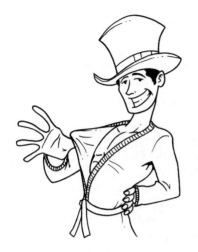

Chapter 15

Out in Style: Right Style, That Is— Movements 1-12

In This Chapter

➤ Learn Kuang Ping movements 1 through 12

➤ What is a "left" style?

➤ Adjusting T'ai Chi to fit your body

➤ How "long Qi" heals when you repulse the monkey

This book can greatly enhance your T'ai Chi experience, offering you value that you may not get otherwise. By fleshing out how and why each movement can benefit you, and understanding the internal mechanics of posture, weight shift, and Qi flow, this book will greatly enrich your T'ai Chi training. You can refer to the following chapters again and again as you learn the forms and movements of T'ai Chi. Since T'ai Chi is constant movement, live classes or video instruction may help you fill in the gaps in the following photographs of T'ai Chi forms. The following chapters, however, will present each movement, numbered as performed in the correct sequence, 1 through 64.

The Kuang Ping Yang style long form takes approximately 20 minutes to complete. This initial form is known as the Right Style. Nearly all the punches will be thrown with the right hand, and most of the movements favor the right side. After learning this 20-minute form, those who really want to dive headlong into T'ai Chi's wonders

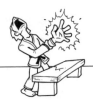

Ouch!

If any of the movement descriptions cause pain, alter them to suit you. For example, on Strike Palm, if you have an injured knee that feels painful when you are asked to put your whole weight on the right leg, then don't put all your weight on your right leg. At that instruction, *put a little more weight on the right,* while still sharing some weight on the left.

might want to learn the Left Style as well. The Left Style is a left-favoring mirror image of the Right Style. So when this section instructs a "right hand" or "right foot" movement, you would move your left hand or foot, and vice versa. You probably want to spend about a year on the initial Right Style before tackling the more advanced Left Style.

Again, for now you are advised to follow the Right Style instructions. The following chapter will take you through the details of the first 12 movements of Kuang Ping Yang Right style. This chapter will get you started with a form you can practice on your own. The *T'ai Chi: Prescription for the Future* video series may be very helpful as well because a fuller explanation of breath, imagery, and relaxation is possible with video. You may also find many excellent T'ai Chi videos, on all the major styles, available through book stores, magazines, or martial arts stores.

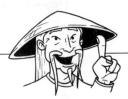

Sage Sifu Says

Remember that the leg your weight shifts to is "filling," while the weight you shift away from is "emptying." They are filling and emptying of both weight and Qi. Enjoying this subtle part of T'ai Chi movement helps to circulate blood and Qi, which is part of its powerful healing process.

Strike Palm to Single Whip

The movement names offer two tools. One is they evoke healthful and soothing mental images to calm the mind and heart. Second, they offer visual mental images to help us remember how to move.

Strike Palm to Ask Blessings, #1

1. Breathe in deeply and lift your palms as if circling them up in front of you over a large three-foot ball, shifting your weight to the left foot.

2. As the palms pull back over the sphere, ending up in front of your chest as though you were going to push something away, the weight shifts back to the right foot, sinking the Qi, or filling the right foot.

3. Your palms drop down to your sides, pulling out and behind your back while rotating out the shoulders. As the empty left foot comes out in front, place the left heel lightly on the ground.

4. Circle your arms around in front of your body as if hugging a large tree, and the left heel touches as your palms meet. The left palm is lateral as in the figure below, while the right palm is vertical. Although the movement is called Strike Palm, the palms don't actually strike; pretend there is a soft energy sphere the size of a honey dew melon between your relaxed, rounded hands.

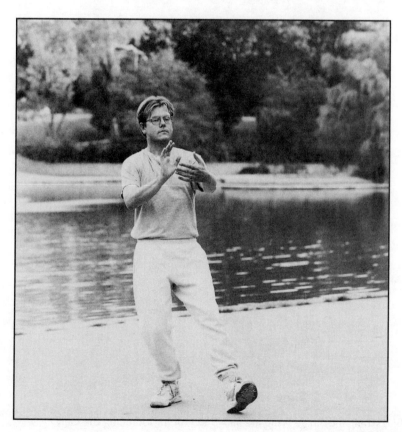

Strike Palm out in front of body.

191

Grasp the Bird's Tail, #2

Stroking the tail down as shifting back.

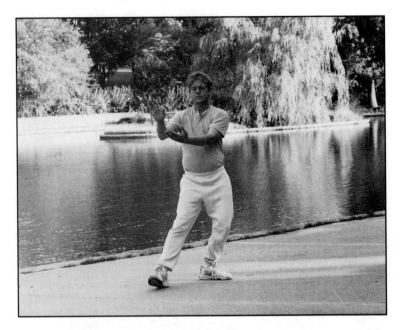

1. With your arms, reach up and out to the right as your left toe reaches out to the left and back.

2. With your right hand palm down on top of your left hand palm up, stroke the bird's tail as your arms pull down and back. Your weight shifts to the left foot behind.

3. Your hands stroke down to the groin, releasing the bird's tail. Turn palms away from your body with your elbows at your sides while your hands continue to circle up in front of your face. Your right foot pulls back touching your right toe near the left instep.

4. Now, turn your dan tien and torso to the right, while your arms follow around and in front of your chest, ready to push out diagonally to right.

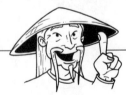

Sage Sifu Says

Strike Palm, Grasp Bird's Tail, and Single Whip are all wonderful for loosening the daily stress from tight shoulders.

Single Whip, #3

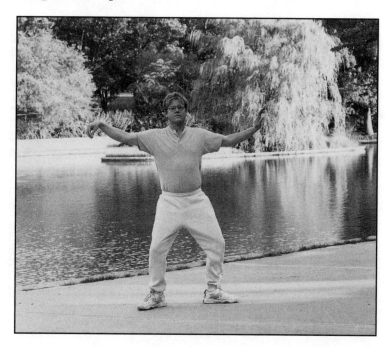

Ducks beak out, full extension, elbow bent.

1. Step out with your right heel, pushing your hands forward as the weight shifts onto the right foot (rolling onto the heel first and then the rest of the foot goes flat).

2. Your arms stretch out to your right side, as the fingers on the right hand bend down to touch your right thumb (forming the Duck's Beak).

3. Your left fingers stroke the inside of the right arm. Your left palm pulls across your body in a great half circle toward the left side as the body follows, turning at the dan tien.

4. Your left palm continues over to the left side, as if circling a globe on its axis, until your palm is near your shoulder and pushes the imaginary globe away to the left, while the weight sinks onto the left heel and then the rest of the left foot.

White Crane Cools to Apparent Closing

The names of these three movements invoke both the peace of nature's calm and the force of martial forms. As with T'ai Chi's philosophy of finding balance, the movements encompass the tenderness and forceful power of movement.

White Crane Cools Its Wings, #4

Straight up and down.

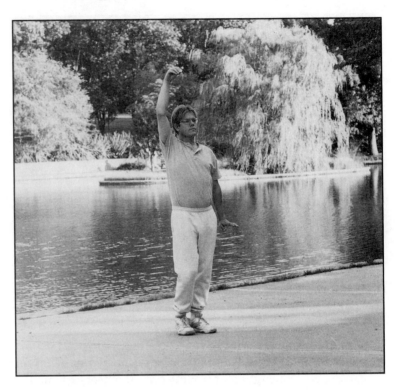

T'ai Sci

Place the tip of the tongue lightly against the roof of the mouth while performing your movements. This changes the structure of the mouth, nose and throat, enabling the breaths to be longer, rather than rapid. Studies show that long, relaxed abdominal breathing oxygenates the body much more effectively than rapidly inflating the chest.

1. Your weight shifts to the left leg as the torso turns to the left. The left arm drops down to your side, the palm facing the ground, as the right arm circles from behind up above head.

2. The right arm comes straight down as the right foot sticks out a few inches in front.

3. Step out to the right side with your right toe.

4. Now, shift the weight to the right foot as the right elbow pulls across in an elbow strike.

5. Lift the left foot and place it out in front, as the left hand moves slightly to the front.

Brush Knee Twist Step, #5

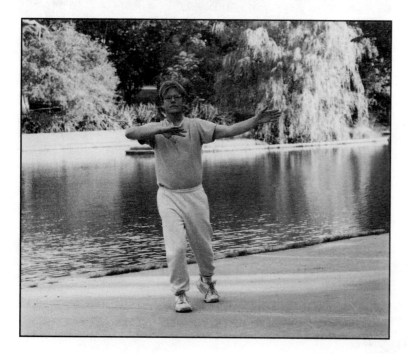

Shifting weight back as arm brushes.

1. The left hand extends out 45 degrees to the left of front, as the left foot steps back behind slightly.

2. Now, the weight sinks back into the left foot as the left arm brushes to the center of the body as if slapping an imaginary wall in front of you.

3. With the weight back on the left foot, the right empty foot steps slightly back as the right hand extends out 45 degrees to the right.

4. Just as you did on the left side, now shift your weight back to the right, brushing the right hand toward your center.

5. Repeat once more on both sides.

6. As you finish the last brush, shift to the right foot and brush across the body with the right hand.

7. Move the left hand out 45 degrees to the left, but do not move the feet.

8. Brush the left hand across the body, and let the left arm circle out in front as the right hand forms a fist by the right hip, before shifting your weight 60 percent onto the left foot and throwing the punch out in front beneath the left arm circling out in a defensive posture, or parry.

Brush Knee Twist Step ends with a parry and punch, which is pictured here for reference, because parry and punches will be performed more later.

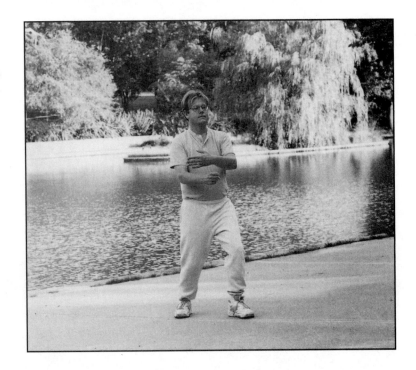

Apparent Closing, #6

Weight on right foot, palms at temples.

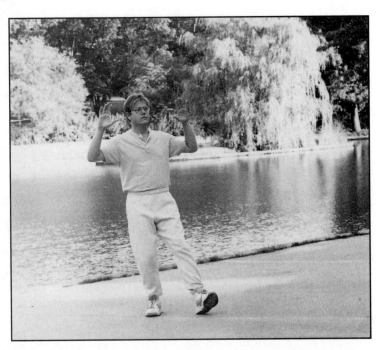

1. From the parry and punch position, the palms turn down, the hands open and come back to the temples, as your weight shifts back onto the right leg and the left foot rolls back on its heel.

2. Push out as the weight rolls forward onto the left leg.

3. Step through with the right foot, and then shift your weight to the right leg as you push out to point with flat hands.

Push to Fist

This section's movements encompass the spiritual images of Focusing Our Mind Toward Our Temple, which is the heart and also our connection to nature with Carry Tiger to Mountain.

Push Turn and Carry Tiger to Mountain, #7

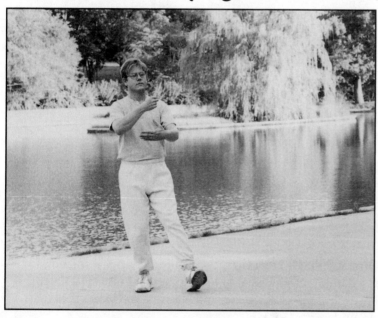

Carry Tiger to Mountain ends with vertical axis aligned over right foot, right fist in front of chest, and left open palm facing abdomen.

1. With your weight on the right foot and your hands pushed out flat, your weight comes off the left foot until only the toe is touching as your pushing hands circle flatly (as if on a table top) to the left as the left foot pivots on the toe.

2. At ¾ of a hand circle, your weight begins shifting to the left foot as the empty right foot pivots on the toe.

3. With the 180-degree turn complete, your weight settles back on the right foot. Only the left heel touches, as your left toes come up off the floor, and your right fist rests over the thumb of your open left hand in front of your abdomen.

Spiraling Hands to Focus Mind Toward the Temple to Parry and Punch, #8

Left heel out, weight in transition and hands about 2 o'clock out to right side in corkscrew.

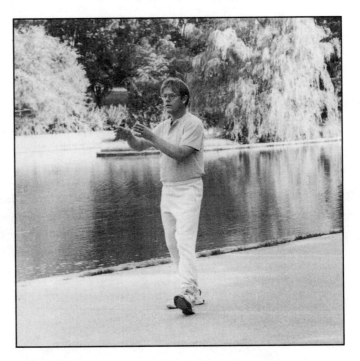

1. With your hands open, the palms should be parallel to one another and pointing straight as the left heel lifts (your weight is still on the right leg) and the left heel lightly retouches the ground.

2. Your weight slowly shifts up to the left foot as your hands begin a clockwise corkscrew. (Keep your hands relaxed at the wrists so that they pivot facing straight.)

3. As your weight shifts completely to the left foot, your hands begin the upward part of a clockwise rotation, lifting the right foot up from behind, as if a string were attached from your hands to your feet, and reaching the top as the right heel touches the ground in front of you.

4. Repeat this with the right foot out this time, and repeat five times, alternating feet.

5. However, on the fifth step, which is with the left foot out, do not shift your weight to the left foot. Leave it out and empty as the hands corkscrew one last time all the way around.

6. Then allow the right hand to fall to your side, forming a fist as the left circles in front to parry.

7. Now, parry and punch with your weight shifting about 65 percent onto the left foot (refer to the previous Brush Knee Twist Step figure).

Fist Under Elbow, #9

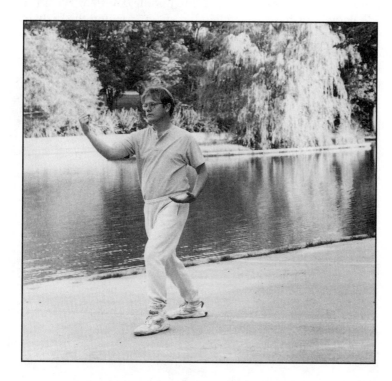

Back fist out with left palm at side.

1. With your weight still mostly on the left foot (in the punch parry position), bring your right fist down under your left elbow.

2. As the right fist is pulled up with the palm facing your chin, the left parry hand drops to the palm up position resting at your left hip.

3. Now, the right fist opens, and the hand relaxes outward.

Repulse to Slanting

This section combines relaxing Traditional Chinese Medicine therapies, powerful martial arts techniques, and exquisitely beautiful dance-like motions.

Repulse the Monkey, #10

Repulse the Monkey can be a powerful martial arts tactic of blocking an incoming blow, yielding to the opponent's force, and allowing that force to carry the opponent flying off to your side. However, it also fosters a very healing exchange of energy,

Traditional Chinese Medicine calls *Long Qi*. During Repulse the Monkey, the open palms pass one another in front of the heart chakra or the middle dan tien. According to Traditional Chinese Medicine, this has a supercharging effect, opening the body to the healing force of the heart dan tien, and practitioners can feel this sense of opening release through that area of the body each time they practice.

Right hand up by shoulder, left hand out ready to push and pull.

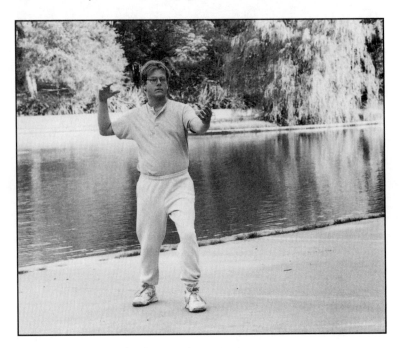

1. Without moving your legs, the left hand (palm up at your waist) begins an outside arc up to the left ear, as if stroking out and away over a large orb at the side of the body.

2. Now the right hand palm up pulls back to the right side of your waist, while the left hand palm facing front pushes outward from your chest; simultaneously, the weight shifts back to the right leg. Prepare for the next three moves by moving the opposite leg back as your palm at waist circles up near the ear, poised to push when the other hand pulls back as you shift back.

3. Repeat with the right hand pushing, the left hand pulling, shifting back to the left leg.

4. Repeat with the left hand pushing, the right hand pulling, shifting back to the right leg.

5. Repeat with the right hand pushing, the left hand pulling, shifting back to the left leg.

Stork Covers Its Wing/Sword in Sheath, #11

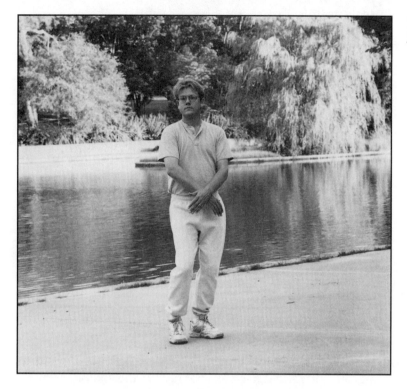

Weight on left, right foot back, hands tucked.

1. With the weight on the left, back foot, the right foot pivots on the heel to follow the extended right arm out diagonally.

2. With the weight shifting to the right foot, pivot on the left ball dropping the left heel in toward the right foot a bit.

3. As the left palm up turns into a sheath, the weight shifts back to the left leg, and the right extended hand pulls back into the left hand's sheath between the left palm and the left hip.

4. The right toe simultaneously pulls back to rest at the left instep.

Slow Palm Slant Flying, #12

Slow Palm Slant Flying is one of the most beautiful and uplifting movements in the entire series.

Fully extended right arm, weight shifting forward to right foot, left foot still down.

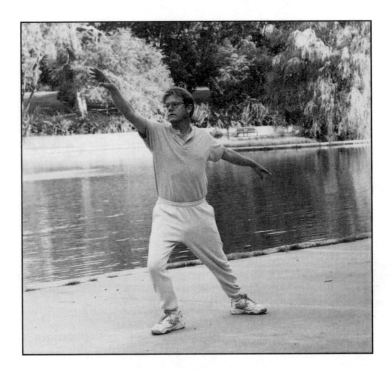

1. The right heel goes out diagonally.

2. Your weight begins to shift to the right foot as the palm extends slowly outward from the left hand's sheath and the left hand extends back to the opposite corner.

3. Extend the arms fully with the weight totally on the right leg; the right arm begins a great arcing circle around your body, while the open left palm arcs up from behind until both open palms meet in front of your chest. Lift the left foot to place the left toe lightly a couple of inches in front of your body below the parallel palms.

The Least You Need to Know

➤ Practice movements with full easy abdominal breaths.

➤ Relax each breath out of the entire body.

➤ Let Qi relax into and through limbs as weight shifts.

➤ Allow yourself to become T'ai Chi's natural elegance.

➤ Long Qi's healing feels great!

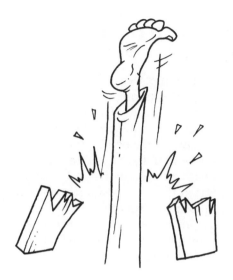

Chapter 16

Kickin' the Light Fantastic— Movements 13–25

In This Chapter

➤ Learn movements 13 through 25

➤ Breathing through life's challenges

➤ Modify kicks to fit you

➤ Moving correctly shifts strain from the lower back to the stronger thighs

---

This chapter will give you an overview of movements 13 through 25 of the Kuang Ping form. Rather than detailing the movements, this chapter will focus on some of the benefits of each movement. Also, you will find helpful insights into the execution of T'ai Chi that will be beneficial, no matter what style you practice.

Raise Right Hand to Fan the Arms

This series of movements encourages a deep release of tension through the entire body. Yet, it also embodies very powerful martial arts applications. T'ai Chi can accomplish the seemingly paradoxical goal of fostering deep relaxation *and* martial arts training, simultaneously.

Ouch!

While moving, remember to breathe deeply into the diaphragm, but also breathe easily and naturally. This conditions us to breathe through life's changes just as we do through T'ai Chi's changing postures.

Raise Right Hand & Left: Turn and Repeat (Part I), #13

Although each movement has powerful martial applications, the goal of T'ai Chi is to "soong yi dien," to loosen up the mind, heart, and body. This movement loosens up the abdominal area by performing Long Qi. In the following figure, you see me pulling my right hand duck's beak up. Prior to that, to form the duck's beak, I reached down with an open right hand passing my left hand which was in the same position as seen in the figure. The palms passing one another healthfully stimulated the dan tien energy center within the body. This is Long Qi. Also, the upper body deeply lets go as the arm is lifted and breath is released.

Although this movement is very soothing to the upper body and therapeutic for the hand and arm, it's martial application is powerful. As the left hand blocks a punch, the right hand lowers to block a kick. The right hand then rises to strike opponent's face or nose, as the right knee raises to kick the groin. Ouch!

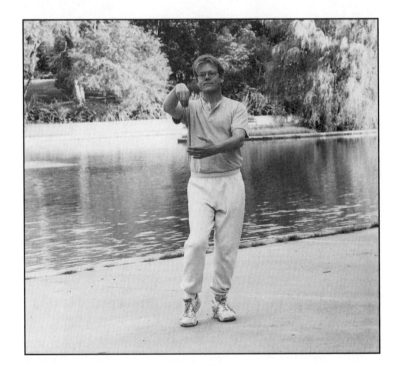

Wave Hand Over Light/Fly Pulling Back, #14

As do many T'ai Chi forms, Fly Pulling Back envisions an orb of energy in front of the body that the hand slips over and then back under, as the body pulls back.

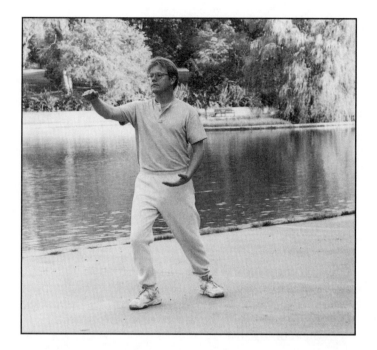

Fly pulling back extends your Qi forward and out in an expressive motion and then relaxes your Qi, sinking back into a retreat.

Fan Through the Arms, #15

The entire body can be allowed to loosen, as the dan tien shifts toward the left leg and the Qi sinks into it. The releasing breath and loosening of the body also allows the energy to flow up and out of the left hand as it relaxes out and away from the body, carried by the force of the dan tien flowing in that direction.

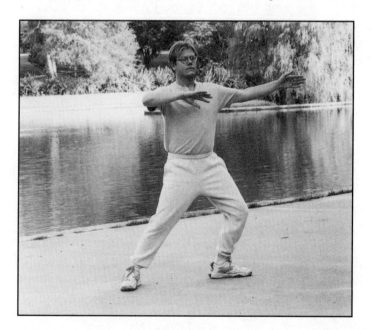

Fan through the arm allows the left arm to relax away from the body as weight shifts towards the left leg. The dan tien is what carries the arm outward, as it shifts over the left leg. The arm moves out and up like a clock hand moving from 6 o'clock to 3 o'clock, as you release a relaxed breath.

Green Dragon to Waving Clouds

These movements are as lovely as the images that describe them. Again, T'ai Chi connects us with nature as we rise up from the water to wave hands like clouds.

Green Dragon Rising from the Water, #16

Green Dragon's shifting weight forward with the hands extended comfortably and slightly upward replicates many motions we perform during the workday or when doing tasks at home, like lifting things onto or off of shelves. By practicing Green Dragon's effortless motion of shifting from the dan tien with proper posture, we establish habits that enable us to move more powerfully in daily tasks, with less exertion and less likelihood of injury.

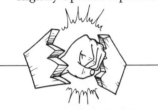

A T'ai Chi Punch Line

During an explanation of how one movement fights off attacks from four different directions, one student wisely explained, "I know where those attacks are coming from now, mostly between here and here" (she said while pointing fingers into each temple of her head). Other people seldom attack us, but our own stress is a frequent assailant. How we handle the world has perhaps more to do with our wellbeing than with how the world handles us. T'ai Chi helps us handle the world's challenges.

Of course there is a martial application as well. The hands extending up can break the grip of an opponent grasping our collar or neck. As you retreat, pull their head down, allowing the force of their attack to pull them off balance.

But again, let T'ai Chi be an effortless flow. There is deep richness to the martial applications of T'ai Chi, but a very healthful way to practice T'ai Chi is to let go of thought. Therefore, you might practice thinking of blows to an opponent sometimes but spend other times simply experiencing the pleasure of movement. Allow the mind and body to flow through the motions effortlessly and soothingly.

When preparing to do Green Dragon Rises, take in a nice full breath and, as you extend up and outward, release the breath in an easy sighing exhale, allowing all the body to let go.

Single Whip (Part II), #17

The Single Whip is aptly named because its motion resembles a whip popping. The hands begin close together over on your right side, then the left hand slides down the forearm, circles around in front of the body, and pushes away to the left like a popping whip. Remember, however, that this is a very slow-motion popping whip.

The full extension of the single whip through the arms can release lots of shoulder tension, as you allow the breath to relax out of the body while the hands extend. It's as if the stress held in the chest, back, and shoulders is being exhaled out through the pushing hand, as the whole body lets go of the breath.

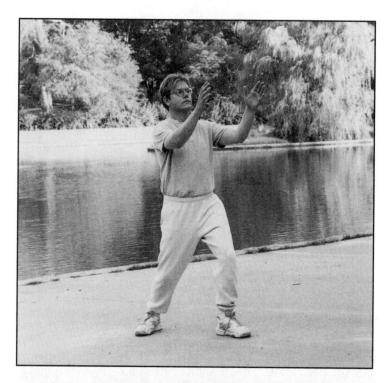

Imagine your hands sliding up the neck of this dragon, slipping around the sides of the dragon's head, and then sliding back down the neck as the body settles back over the back foot.

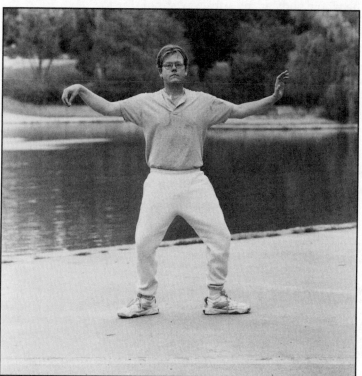

The right hand drops the duck's beak, with all the fingers on the right hand extending down to touch the right thumb. Modern carpal tunnel prevention exercises include exercises like these. So, among its many benefits, T'ai Chi appears to be an ergonomic carpal tunnel prevention exercise as well.

Wave Hands Like Clouds (X 3), #18 (Part I, Linear Style)

In Wave Hands Like Clouds, the lead arm is always in an elbow strike position, while the trailing hand drops down to protect the groin.

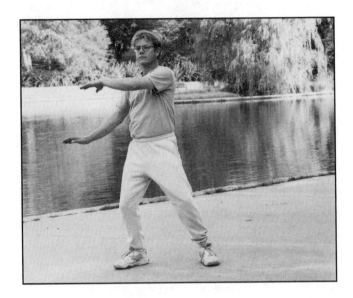

Even though this is obviously martial in application, there is also the soothing quality of imagining the hands waving like clouds. The thought unlocks an effortless quality that can flow through the whole body as the arms wave from side to side.

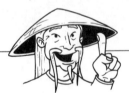

Sage Sifu Says

T'ai Chi is taught in three stages. First, the movements are learned. Second, the breath is incorporated into the regimen by learning an inhalation or exhalation that is connected to each movement. Thirdly, a relaxation element or awareness of the flow of energy through the body is learned. Although the first step offers many benefits from the first day, the benefits get richer and deeper with each level you learn.

Single Whip to Separate Foot

This series completes with the initial kicks. These lovely movements are performed differently by each practitioner. But, no matter how high or low *your* kicks are, this will be great for balance and coordination.

Single Whip (Part III), #19

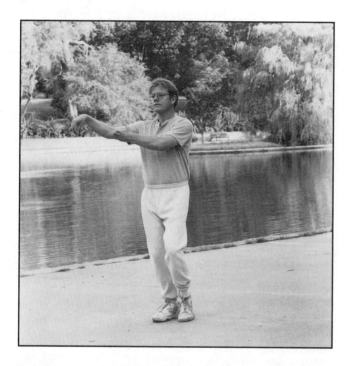

Before the single whip extends out as in movement #17 shown previously, the left hand slides down the right forearm as in this figure, before then circling around in front of the body.

High Pat on Horse/Guarding the Temples, #20

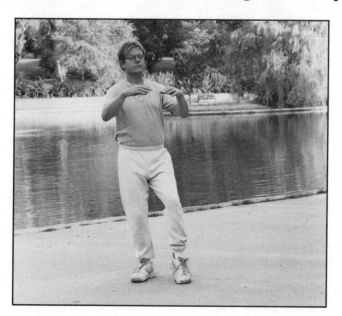

The hands pat an imaginary horse's behind, at about heart level in front. Simultaneously, the toe touches slightly out in front of the body.

Lower Block/Upper Block, Separation of Right Foot; Lower Block/Upper Block, Separation of Left Foot, #21

When kicking or separating the right foot, the right wrist is crossed over the left wrist in front of the groin. Then the wrists, still crossed, rise up to chest level and twist outward to block up slightly above the head.

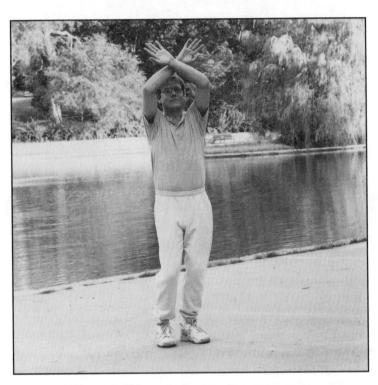

Ouch!

Remember there is no correct height to kick at. Your kick may be only a few inches off the ground, or, if you're a soccer player, your kick may be two feet higher than in the figure for movement #22. There is no wrong or right. The only rule is that you relax and enjoy yourself. So, trying to kick higher than feels good is against the rules. As you practice over days and months, your kicks will effortlessly get higher.

As the right leg is kicked up on the right side, the right hand arches out and over to touch the pinky side of the right hand on the kicking foot. Your hand may not touch at first. That's okay; just kick as high as is comfortable.

Kick with Sole to Double Kick

The kick sequence gets more beautiful through this series. Wind Blowing Lotus Leaves not only soothes the body and mind, but can also help your body learn to push the lawn mower with less pressure on your lower back. Correct T'ai Chi movement shifts the strain from your lower back to your thighs. Our thighs are much stronger, and the femur is much less delicate than our back's vertebrae.

Turn and Kick with Sole, #22

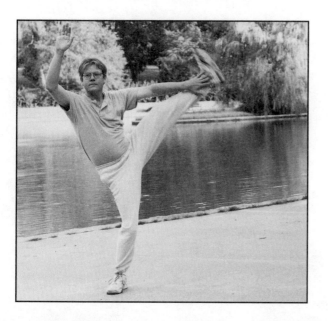

Rather than striking out and down with the hand as in Separation Kicks, on this kick, the hand slides out in front of the body from the block and arcs back in to slap near the instep of the left foot.

Wind Blowing Lotus Leaves (X 4), #23

This is an exquisite move. It's artistically beautiful and feels fantastic because it loosens the entire torso. As you shift forward slightly turning the body, the breath relaxes out of every cell. As your Qi sinks into the earth, its power also flows through you and out your hands. Therefore the power of the push is from the dan tien and not the shoulder. This is better for your back.

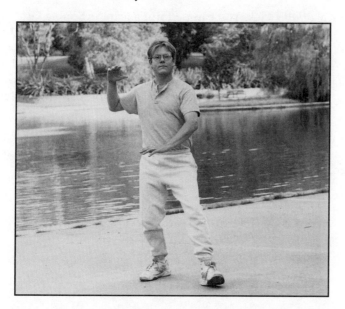

As you relax your weight forward onto the front foot, the back foot stays flat. The back arm really doesn't move, following in place as the body shifts forward. The front hand drops down in a groin block.

211

Block Up/Fist Down, #24

Be sure not to lean forward as you strike with the hammer fist. Posture, as always, is comfortably aligned above the dan tien.

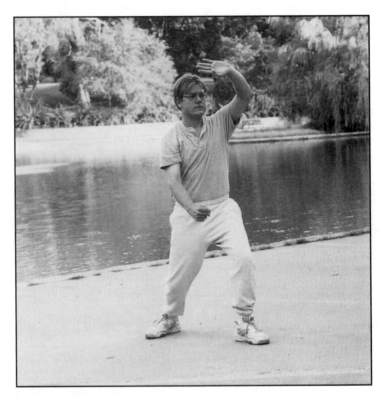

Turn & Double Kick, #25

There are two ways to do the double kick. You can perform a leaping double kick whereby you scissor-kick your legs; while the left leg is still up in the air, kick up the right leg while bringing down the left leg to land. Followed by placing the right foot down in front and shifting forward onto it. Or, you can use the lower impact double kick exhibited in the following figure. Kick the left leg up in front, then place it down and shift your weight to it before the right leg is kicked up and slapped with the right palm striking down.

Either kick is beautiful and energizing; however, the second is much lower impact and recommended for those using T'ai Chi as therapy. Remember your kick does not have to be as high as illustrated.

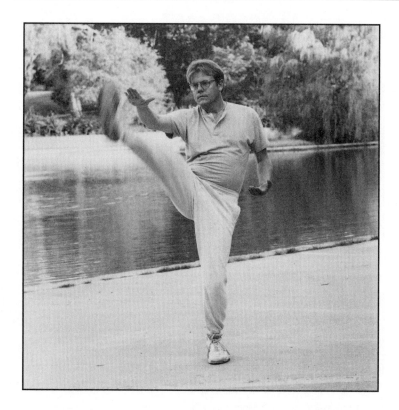

As the right leg kicks up, the right palm turns over and smacks down to slap the top of the right foot, or calf, or knee, or wherever your hand comfortably slaps without leaning forward.

The Least You Need to Know

➤ T'ai Chi's powerful self-defense moves can be soothing.

➤ Breathe fully and easily throughout all movements.

➤ Feel at one with the world when practicing.

➤ Push from your dan tien, not your shoulders or back.

➤ Most battles are fought in our own minds and hearts, and this is where T'ai Chi works its magic.

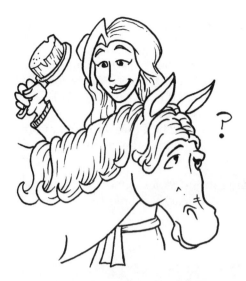

Chapter 17

Part a Wild Horse's Mane— Movements 26–38

In This Chapter

➤ Learn movements 26 through 38

➤ Learn how to relax while boxing with four opponents

➤ Learn how to combine power with effortless motion

➤ Learn practical movement therapies with a dancer's elegance

---

This chapter illustrates some of the most beautiful T'ai Chi moves. Each one provides tremendous improvements in balance, posture, coordination, and grace. Of course, there is powerful therapeutic value in each one as well. The information in this chapter is helpful to inspire you to begin practicing T'ai Chi, but once you start, the powerful benefits will come *effortlessly*.

Parry/Punch to Separate Foot

This section's movements are martial, yet useful for practical everyday life. The punches teach pushing with less back strain, while the standing kick improves balance.

Ouch!

Never force or strain. Breathe easily. Let your mind and body learn to relax as you are absorbed in the silken flow of continuous movement.

Parry & Punch, #26

Although most T'ai Chi movements have martial applications, none is as obvious as Parry & Punch. As the punch is thrown and the Qi sinks into the forward left leg, the breath is released in an easy sigh. This action is a wonderful stress release for both the hips and the upper body. Tension can be allowed to pour out the left foot into the earth, and upper body tension can be released out the punching fist.

Again, do not lean forward as you punch. The body or vertical axis always stays stacked above the dan tien.

From the double kick, the right foot is put down in front. Shift on to it, step forward with left foot, dropping the left arm in front as pictured, and punching out with the right fist from right hip. Do not lean forward.

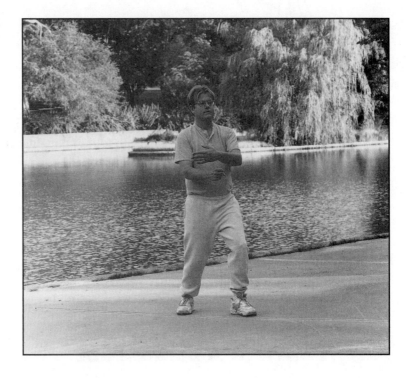

216

Step Back/Lower Block/Upper Block; Kick Front, #27

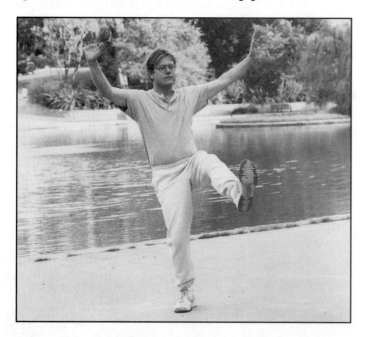

This kick is great for balance. You do not have to perform the kick this high. You may begin much lower. Go as high as is comfortable, without leaning backwards out of your vertical axis. As with all movements it is done very slowly, placing the foot out in front as you breathe and observe your balance.

Lower Block/Upper Block Separation of Right Foot, #28

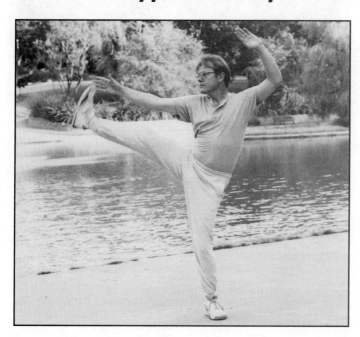

Cross wrists at groin to block low, raise crossed wrists to block at face, and then twist wrists out to block up. Kick out right foot and separate foot by arcing right hand out. Always kick only as high as is comfortable. Some practitioners only kick a few inches high, but they are moving, growing, loosening, and improving each time they do it.

Do not psyche yourself into thinking this isn't for you. It is perfect for you. If you are in a wheelchair, this movement will involve your hand arcing down. If you are paralyzed to the waist, you will give the right side abdominal muscles instructions to extend upward toward the arcing right hand, and this intention of motion will exercise and coordinate mind and body, while relieving tension.

Parry/Punch to Sink to Earth

These movements will integrate upper body force with the power of hip and dan tien rotation. They also beautifully integrate yielding with impending force, as in Sink to the Earth.

Parry & Punch, #29

Notice that as the punch begins, the weight is still on the back foot, while the front foot is empty. This is because the power of the punch comes from the dan tien shifting from one foot to the other. The fist is just an extension of the moving dan tien.

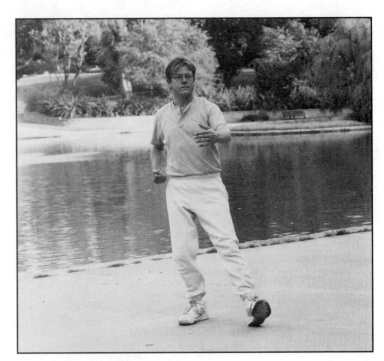

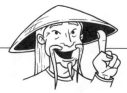

Sage Sifu Says

When punching or pushing in T'ai Chi, remember that these martial exercises can also be about how we move through our lives: cutting the grass, washing the dishes, or putting groceries in the pantry. If we adopt good postural habits by moving from the dan tien and vertical axis while punching or pushing, then we will likely use these habits while mowing or lifting groceries out of the trunk of the car.

Chop Opponent with Fist (Pivot & Rotate Fist (X 3), #30

Turn around fully, or 180 degrees, from Parry & Punch before beginning Chop Opponent. When turning, you must empty a leg before pivoting on it. That way, you do not damage the knee. Once a foot is pivoted to the desired position, then weight can be returned to it.

Sink to the Earth/Backward Elbow Strike, #31

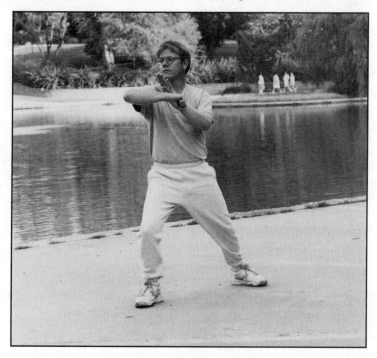

Chop Opponent involves an elbow strike stepping to the right, a punch stepping to the left, and an elbow strike stepping to the right.

When doing elbow striking behind, do not feel you must go this low. The depth of this strike is all in the bend of the left knee. If your knee only feels comfortable with a slight bend, then that is perfect for you.

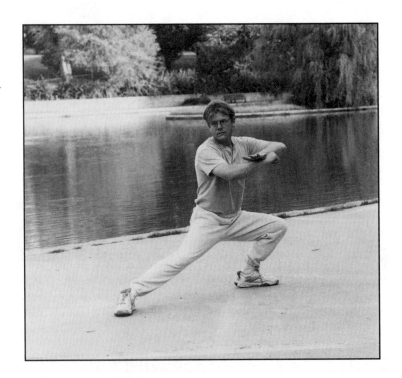

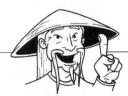

Sage Sifu Says

Many of our problems come from mindlessly forcing ourselves to live in ways that do not feel good to us. As T'ai Chi teaches us to move in the ways that feel good to us, rather than forcing our body to do it the way the teacher or the person next to us moves, we learn to "listen." Listening to what feels right is the most powerful thing we can do for ourselves and for our world. This is the essence of T'ai Chi.

Single Whip to Fair Lady

This section is incredibly beautiful and yet powerfully martial in application. These motions can build grace in the dancer and unleash power in the boxer.

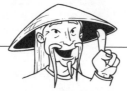

Sage Sifu Says

The complexity and variety of movements may seem daunting at first, but just relax and learn the move you're learning today. You'll get it, one move at a time.

Single Whip, ³/₄ Single Whip (Part IV), #32

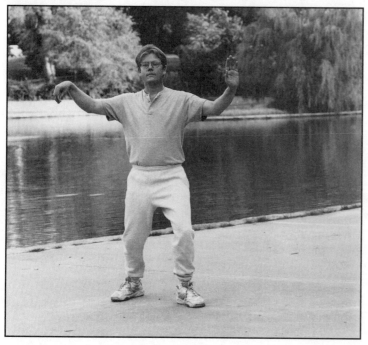

From the elbow strike behind, we turn forward, and punch up at a 45-degree angle out to the right. From this punch we turn, drop our duck's beak out to the right, and begin the single whip—only this single whip is finished out at a 45-degree angle to the left.

Partition of Wild Horse's Mane (X4) & Single Whip, #33

Strike out left, right, left, and right, before going into another full Single Whip. Parting the Wild Horse's Mane is a lot like Wave Hands Like Clouds, except Wave Hands Like Clouds goes sideways, while Partition of Horse's Mane goes at 45-degree angles forward.

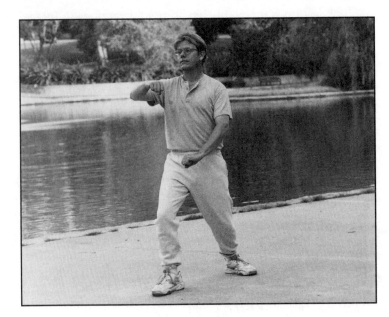

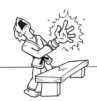

Ouch!

On all pushes, strikes, and punches, the back foot stays down until the front foot is completely full and the push or punch is complete. If you raise the back foot as you strike, the only thing behind that strike is a wobbly little ankle. However, if the back foot stays down, you have the whole planet behind it.

Fair Lady Works at Shuttles, #34

Fair Lady Works at Shuttles is actually a shadow boxing routine involving blocks and punches used to spar with four opponents coming from four different directions.

➤ Pivot; Defend; Punch Left

➤ Defend; Punch Right

➤ Pivot; Defend; Punch Left

➤ Defend; Punch Right Through

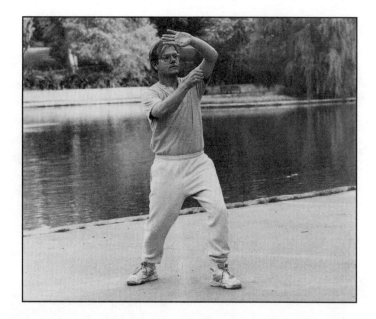

Again, note that before pivoting to the next movement, the back foot remains down flat until the punch is complete. This places the entire planet behind your punch, and with the body in a state of "song" or relaxation, the force of the earth flows up through your body.

Grasping Tails to Return to Earth

This section unites us with the lovely ebbs and flows of the natural world. Caressing the Bird's Tail, Waving Hands Like Clouds, and then returning these cosmic experiences to the solid roots of earth, in Return to Earth.

Grasp the Bird's Tail (Part II), #35

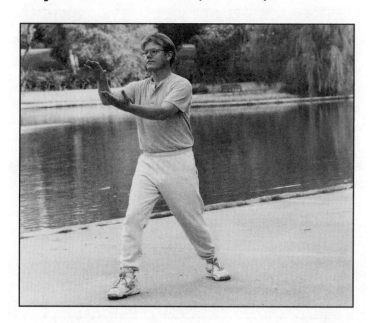

This is the same as the first Grasp the Bird's Tail, except to get in position you step forward from the last punch of Fair Lady Works at Shuttles with your right foot out to grasp bird's tail.

Single Whip (Part V), #36

Notice how the left hand circles around the imaginary globe off to the left on Single Whips.

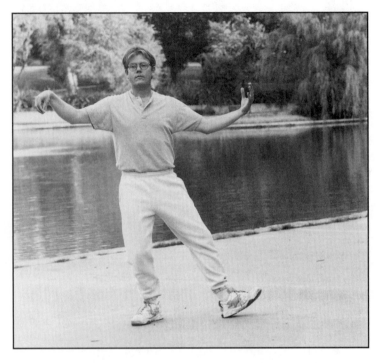

Wave Hands Like Clouds (Part II, Linear Style), #37

As the arms pull across the front of your body and the weight shifts, exhale in a relaxed natural breath. When your arms are switching off to the right or left, and you are moving a leg into position, inhale.

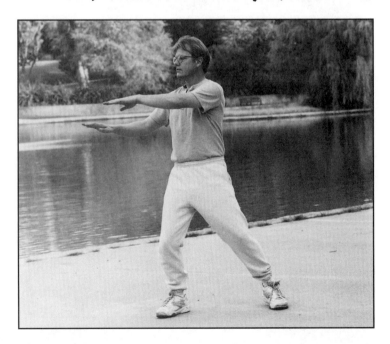

Incorporating breath with each movement slows down the movement and makes it a relaxing and centering exercise, of and by itself. When doing T'ai Chi, you are never doing the entire form in your mind, for your mind is always absorbed on the movement you are on *right now*. This helps the mind and emotions practice the art of *focus*.

Single Whip Down; Return to the Earth (Part I), #38

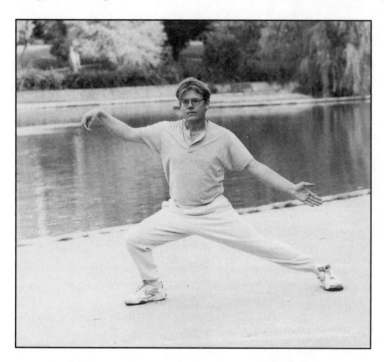

As the left hand circles around to the left, the left foot extends out to the left, touching first the toe, then the foot fills somewhat. Now, the right knee bends and the body sinks into the right foot as pictured. Do not bend over, the depth is determined by the right knee's bend. Only go as low as feels good to you. There is no right depth, except what is right for you.

The Least You Need to Know

➤ Remember T'ai Chi is *effortless.*

➤ Adjust movements to fit your mobility.

➤ Doing movements correctly teaches your body to lift groceries correctly.

➤ Pushing and punching with the back foot planted and the body relaxed guides the force of the earth through you.

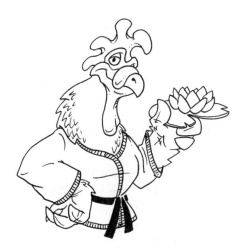

Chapter 18

From Golden Cock to Water Lily—Movements 39–51

In This Chapter

➤ Learn movements 39 through 51

➤ Why posture can energize or exhaust you

➤ Relax while boxing opponent's ears

➤ Learn the crescent kick

At first, movements may look too physically demanding. However, the creators of T'ai Chi were very aware of how our bodies work and remember that T'ai Chi was originally designed for out-of-shape monks. So, as you learn the movements presented in previous chapters, that learning prepares your body for the subsequent movements. By the time you get to these movements, your balance and posture will be different from when you began T'ai Chi. In fact, *you will be different*. Your nervous system and skeletal/muscular systems will be functioning at a higher, more integrated level.

For those who are more athletic or for those with physical limitations, don't feel left out. Even a top athlete will benefit from the advancing complexity of these movements, in both balance and overall dexterity. For those with physical limitations, you will simply modify these forms in a way that works for you. Kicks can be lower or nonexistent if you're in a wheelchair. Even if you only have motion in one arm or just the neck and head, then that is the part of the movement you will practice. T'ai Chi is for everyone, *especially you*. Remember that T'ai Chi is a celebration of movement. *Whatever movement* you are able to perform can be a soothing relaxation therapy when incorporated with mindful motion, full slow breaths, and a feeling of effortless release.

Before moving on to the next set of movements, try this: Standing comfortably in the Horse Stance, close your eyes and breathe while relaxing the entire body. Standing in your proper vertical axis with the head stacked up above the lower dan tien, you can let the body almost completely relax.

Now, lean your head forward (with eyes still closed), noticing how the muscles must tighten to hold you up. Let the head go back into vertical axis alignment and notice how effortless the stance becomes. Now, lean the head back a few inches and notice the tightening up of the muscles throughout the body to hold you up. Golden Cock to Stork's Wing

Moving in vertical axis posture will make everything more effortless. Practicing T'ai Chi with this awareness of effortless versus effortful movement will easily and naturally change the way you move through life.

Golden Cock Stands on One Leg (X 4), #39

The hand pushes out at the same time the leg kicks out. Do not kick out so high that you lean back. Remember always to maintain vertical axis; this balance allows the movement to be effortless.

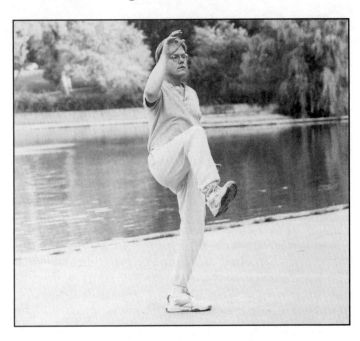

This series of movements is great fun. Although they look demanding in terms of balance, if you've learned the movements leading up to this, you'll be amazed how easily you will do them. You probably didn't realize how much T'ai Chi has already improved your balance.

Repulse the Monkey (X 3) (Part II), #40

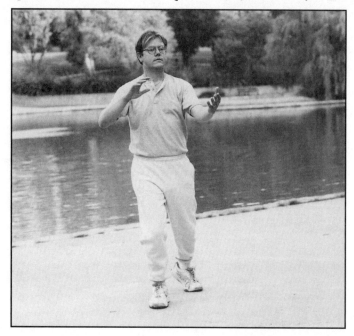

As you push the right hand out and pull the left hand back, the palms will pass each other somewhere in front of the heart. Traditional Chinese Medicine calls this crossing of the palms Long Qi. It energizes the chakra, or energy center, nearest to the Long Qi.

You should repeat Repulse the Monkey three times. Each time you practice Repulse the Monkey, you may notice a distinct "letting go" in the chest, heart, and upper-back area.

When stepping backward for Repulse the Monkey, do not "walk the tight-rope" by placing your retreating foot directly behind the other foot. When you place the foot behind, place it slightly out to the side, making some space between your legs. This will make balance much easier when walking backward.

Stork Covers Its Wing/Sword in Sheath (Part II), #41

From the last Repulse the Monkey, the right arm pulls back to the left hip as the left hand turns in to form a sheath between the hip and hand for the right hand to slip into. The right foot comes back to touch at instep of the left foot.

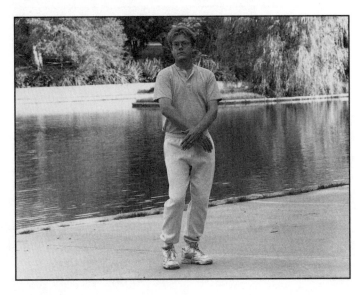

Palm Slanting to Fly Pulling Back

These motions offer deep muscular releases of shoulder and back tension. Also, our tendency to lean out of our "vertical axis" is corrected as these movements help us become more aware of our postural habits.

Slow Palm Slant Flying (Part II), #42

Stepping out with the right heel, you then extend out your arms as seen in the figure. This movement is a powerful release of upper body tension, while opening the mind, heart, and body to a much greater sense of energy as the tension is released.

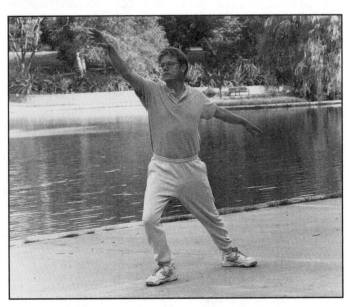

There is also a sense of physical solidity and power experienced through this exquisitely artistic movement.

Raise Right & Left Hands; Turn & Repeat (Part II), #43

Refer to Chapter 16, movement #13 for figures of Raise Right & Left Hands. That same movement is repeated here.

Wave Hand Over Light/Fly Pulling Back, #44

Refer to Chapter 16, movement #14 for figures of Wave Hand Over Light/Fly Pulling Back. That same movement is repeated here.

Arm Fanning Through Single Whip

Just as Fanning Through the Arm allows deep tension releases through the hips, Box Opponent's Ears can foster releases through the spine, shoulders, and head.

Fan Through the Arm (Backhand Slap), #45

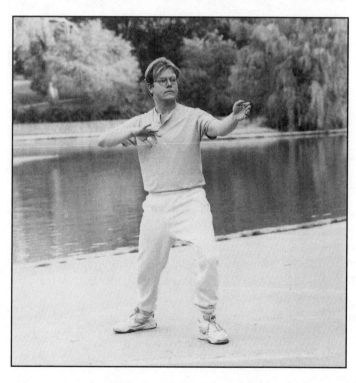

This backhand slap is performed almost exactly as movement #15 in Chapter 16, with one slight difference. In #15, the left hand fans up the left side to shoulder height, as a clock hand would go from 6 o'clock to 9 o'clock. However, in movement #45, the left hand flows out in front of your body around to the left side, as if you were striking someone to your left with a backhanded slap.

Step Push/Box Opponent's Ears/ Cannon Through Sky, #46

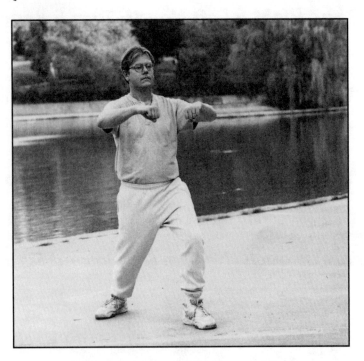

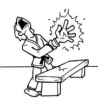

Ouch!

Make sure not to "lean" into your opponent as you box ears. Remember all punches come from shifting the dan tien forward, rather than from a lunging upper body.

This series is a powerful advancing attack involving three rapid consecutive blows:

1. This movement begins with the right foot stepping forward, while shifting to it as you push away in front.

2. Step forward again with the right foot and Box Opponent's Ears.

3. Step forward again with the right foot, back fist striking with right hand, while placing left fist on muscle of right forearm.

Single Whip (Part VI), #47

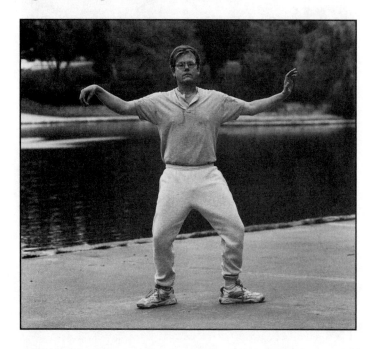

The Single Whip loosens the back, shoulders, and chest muscles to foster an open flow of Qi throughout the upper body. This movement can help increase breathing capacity and is great for easing asthma or emphysema.

Waving Clouds to Water Lily Kick

Beginning with soothing cloud waving, this section culminates in the crescent kick, or Cross Wave of Water Lily Kick. These moves deeply loosen both upper and lower body.

Wave Hands Like Clouds (Round Style; Part I), #48

Circular, or Round, Style Wave Hands Like Clouds is an exquisite movement. It loosens the entire body if done with smooth easy breaths and your awareness centered in the dan tien. As you move the loosening of Qi, energy permeates all the tissue of the body through the macrocosmic cycle of all the energy meridians.

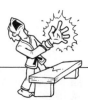

Ouch!

Beware of the "creeping butt syndrome." If Wave Hands Like Clouds ever causes lower back pain, you are probably allowing your sacral vertebrae (or butt) to creep out behind you, causing you to over-arch your lower back. Each time you let a breath out, allow the lower back muscles to relax and the tailbone to drop. Do not force it down, let it relax down.

This is performed just as the earlier linear form of Wave Hands Like Clouds, except the palms face into the body rather than down to the ground. Pretend you are holding a great soap bubble, lightly enough not to pop it, but keeping it from spilling over the side or slipping down through your rounded arms.

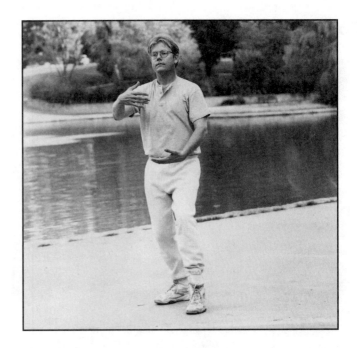

Single Whip (Part VII), #49

This is a repetition of Movement #47.

High Pat on Horse (Part II), #50

From the Single Whip, the left hand stays in place as the right arm circles around. Once the right arm is around, both arms bend and relax like a horseshoe, before patting the horse's behind in front. Shift your weight back to the right foot, as the left toe touches out front.

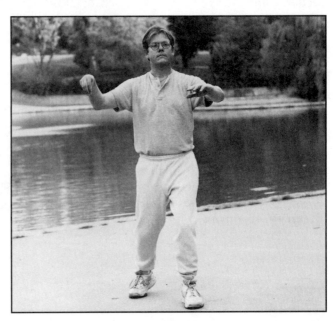

Cross Wave of Water Lily Kick (Part I), #51

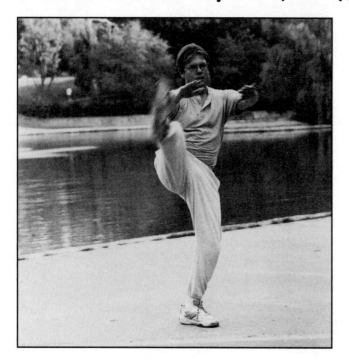

Shifting to the left foot, the right leg kicks to the left and pulls across in a clockwise motion to form a crescent kick. Simultaneously, both flat hands, palms down, circle up and around clockwise to lightly slap the top of the right foot as they meet, as shown in the figure.

Remember you can't get your kicks when straining. Your kicks may only be a few inches off the ground, and your hands may touch your thigh rather than your foot. The main thing is to do the kick in a way that is comfortable for you. This way it is fun, and you will continue without injury to improve over time.

The Least You Need to Know

➤ Each movement learned and practiced transforms you.

➤ The good relaxed posture taught by T'ai Chi is power.

➤ No matter how expansive or limited your mobility, T'ai Chi extends it.

➤ Don't force yourself to increase mobility. Let it effortlessly blossom over time.

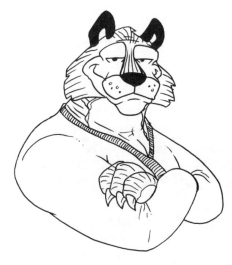

Chapter 19

Ain't It Grand? Terminus, That Is— Movements 52–64

In This Chapter

➤ Learn movements 52 through 64

➤ Use T'ai Chi to help prevent repetitive stress injuries

➤ Relax into "complexity"

➤ How to tap into universal, limitless energy

Congratulations! You deserve a great deep bow. Upon completion of learning the entire 64 posture series of the Kuang Ping Yang style form, you get to do the most wonderful movement of all, Grand Terminus. This final move cleanses and reinvigorates the body, leaving you feeling about *as terrific as a kid could feel,* or as Dave Letterman might say, *"Feeling better than people should be allowed."*

Grand Terminus is not only the last T'ai Chi movement, it is also the name of that popular yin/yang symbol you see on jewelry. The white wave interacting with the black wave symbolizes a balance of all things, hard and soft, force and yielding, concentration and empty awareness. Each time you complete your T'ai Chi forms, you will have integrated all aspects of yourself. You will have centered yourself in all ways. The Grand Terminus is a completion of renewal and a gateway to greater and greater adventures. As you learn to move smoothly and effortlessly through an increasingly meaningful life, an ancient friend called T'ai Chi will always be there to console and inspire, no matter what life throws at you.

Strike Down to Single Whip

This series of movements has a strong martial application, but each movement also challenges us to relax even when using force.

Parry Up; Downward Strike, #52

As you punch downward, try not to bend your back over. Again, we always maintain our vertical axis, aligning the three dan tien points vertically.

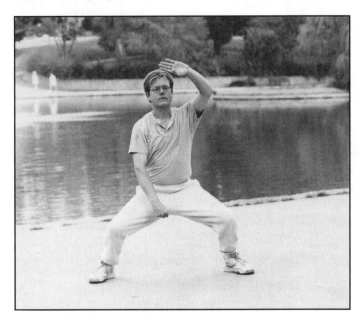

Grasp the Bird's Tail (Part III), #53

As a martial movement, Grasp the Bird's Tail is about yielding to the force of an incoming punch, helping its forward momentum with a pull as your weight shifts back, thereby allowing the opponent to hurtle past you.

The health benefits of Grasp the Bird's Tail are equal to its martial effectiveness. Breathe in as hands reach out and relax the breath out as the hands pull back. This, plus relaxing the muscles around the rib cage, increases breathing capacity. Also, the half rotation of shoulders and full rotation of elbows may be effective therapy to help avoid the plague of repetitive stress injuries that many peoples' jobs cause.

Single Whip (Part VIII), #54

This movement is a repetition of Movement #47 in Chapter 18.

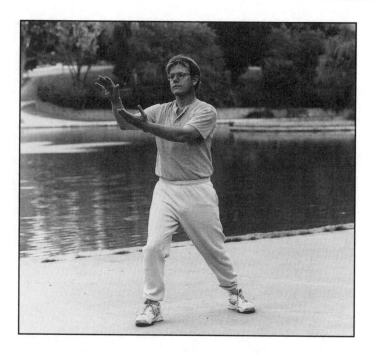

This Grasp the Bird's Tail is a bit different because you step up with your right foot to grab the tail, rather than stepping back with your left foot.

Waving Clouds to Seven Stars

Beginning with the gentle flow of clouds, we culminate this section with a powerful blow. The Single Whip Down allows us to test our mobility slowly and gently.

Wave Hands Like Clouds (Round Style; Part II), #55

See Movement #48, Chapter 18; this is a repetition of it.

On Wave Hands Like Clouds, remember that the leg moves as the hands move away from the centerline of the body. When the hands pull into the centerline, the weight is shifting. Breathe in when the hands reach away from the centerline and exhale when the weight shifts, relaxing the weight and sinking the Qi into the filling leg.

Single Whip Down; Return to the Earth (Part II), #56

Single Whip Down can be modified with a slight bend of the right knee. Go to a depth of comfort. Let the depth of the knee bend descend over a period of months and years. There is no horse race with T'ai Chi. Take comfort in the fact that while others get stiffer as they age, you are getting more supple and flexible.

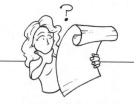

Know Your Chinese

Other ancient styles refer to **Single Whip Down** as *Snake Creeps Down*.

Do not lean over when doing Single Whip Down; the spine stays erect. The depth of Single Whip Down is determined by bending your right knee. You sink your Qi into the right leg.

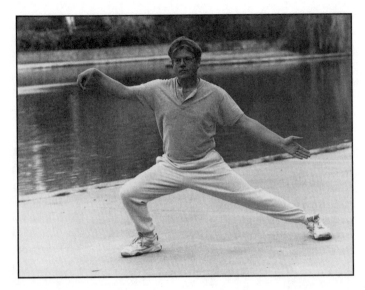

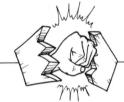

A T'ai Chi Punch Line

Some students theorize that when the opponent experiences the groin level punch of Form Seven Stars, they "see seven stars."

Step Up to Form Seven Stars, #57

Form Seven Stars connects you to the universe by punching the right fist in a down and upward arc toward the heavens.

Right fist punches up at groin level. Try to keep back erect, without leaning too much.

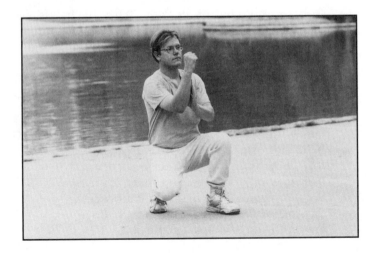

Retreating Tiger to Water Lily Kick

The complexity of this series is at first a bit mind-boggling. However, as that complexity is absorbed into our being, we grow from it, and that growth feels great! The difficulty of learning complex movements, coupled with the QiGong relaxation exercises incorporated into T'ai Chi practice teaches us how to relax even as our mind absorbs complex information. This not only feels good but in a way stretches our mind's capacity to comprehend, absorb, and function. This ability carries over into all aspects of our lives.

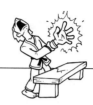

Ouch!

Step Up to Form Seven Stars does not have to be done with knees bent as much as in the figure above. The height of stance or depth of knee bend as always is determined by your comfort. Many do this with only a slight bending of the knees, standing almost completely erect.

Retreat to Ride the Tiger, #58

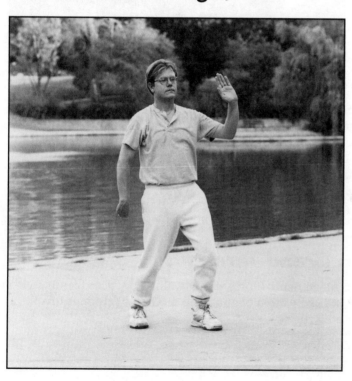

As you block out with the left hand, the right forms a duck's beak behind. Do not let the left leg straighten out. This puts pressure on joints. T'ai Chi is done with the elbows and knees always slightly bent.

Slanting Body/Turn the Moon, #59

Although these blocks have very direct martial applications, they are soothing to the upper body. Breathe easily and enjoy the circular movement of the right arm blocking up and out, while the left hand arcs easily down to form the duck's beak behind. As you memorize the movements, such as this one, the silken flowing will be more and more soothing each time you perform it.

As the right hand blocks out and the left hand forms the duck's beak behind, the left toe touches lightly in front.

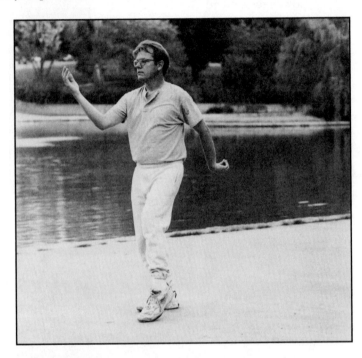

Cross Wave of Water Lily (Part II), #60

This movement is a repetition of movement #51 in Chapter 18.

Shooting Tiger to Grand Terminus

This section's movements blend martial force with yielding flow. This blend of yin and yang motion is invited to fill every atom of our being, as Grand Terminus invokes a universe of life energy to pour through us.

Stretch Bow to Shoot Tiger, #61

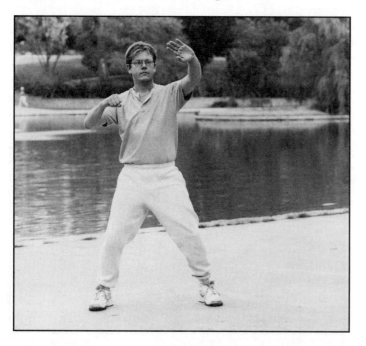

Imagine you are stretching a bow string back with the right hand, while the left hand aims the bow out to the left at a 45-degree angle. The right hand will settle at the right hip before punching out around and to the center. Then the left hand punches out and around, while the right hand returns to the hip. Both hands punch and return for five punches, beginning with the right fist and ending with the right fist.

Grasp the Bird's Tail (Right Style), #62

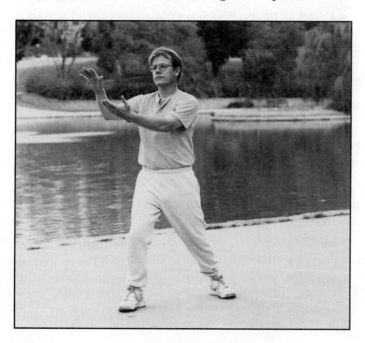

Perform a standard Grasp the Bird's Tail movement and then reach forward out to the right/front at 45 degrees. As if you were holding the moon delicately in your hands, retreat your weight to the back foot. Imagine the moonlight's healing essence spilling over your head and body, as the hands pull back toward your body.

Grasp the Bird's Tail (Left Style), #63

This is the only left style movement in these 64 postures. Step back with the right foot, this time reaching out to the front left. Relax as the weight settles back and the moonlight pours over your loosening body.

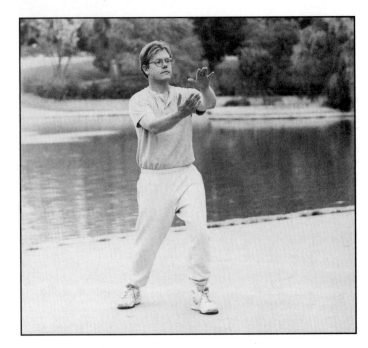

Grand Terminus; Gather Heaven to Earth, #64

This movement is meant to gather all the light, or Qi, we have generated through the 64 movements. As the hands turn downward at the top of their arcs, allow the light to spill, washing over and through your entire being to cleanse any heavy loads or toxins. Let the feet open to release any loads right down into the earth's gentle pull. Continue to allow the light to wash over and through you throughout the day.

1. The hands reach out and slightly back, extending the arms back and outward.

2. As you stretch up, the knees straighten for the first time throughout the entire 64 posture series.

3. Gathering the Qi from all around, the light pours over your relaxing body as the palms turn down.

4. Slowly, the palms descend, invoking the cleansing light to wash through every area as the palms pass through.

5. As the hands descend back to your sides, just bask in the soothing healing of this ocean of light washing over and through. Experience effortlessness.

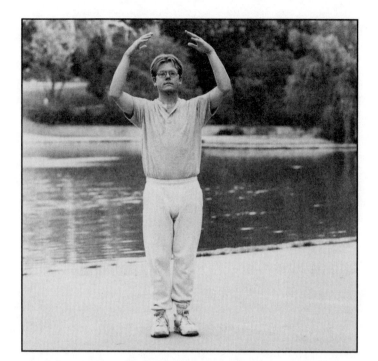

"EXPERIENCE the Light!"

The Least You Need to Know

➤ T'ai Chi leaves you fully integrated and invigorated.

➤ T'ai Chi is a physical way to practice "rolling with life's punches."

➤ T'ai Chi connects you to the heaven and earth.

➤ T'ai Chi practices letting go of what's inevitable, and diving into what's changeable.

Part 5

T'ai Chi's Buffet of Short, Sword and Fan Styles

About a mere 30 years ago there was almost no T'ai Chi available to Westerners. T'ai Chi was a Chinese secret. However, today we are fortunate to live in interesting times, as the Chinese would say.

In most cities today you can find a variety of T'ai Chi styles, including not only basic forms, but the more artistic and challenging sword and fan styles, as well. Feast your eyes on just a sampling of the wide variety of short forms, sword style, and fan style T'ai Chi now available to you, and then choose an adventure to embark upon.

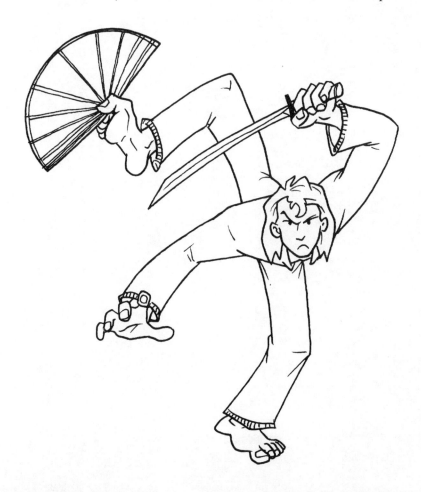

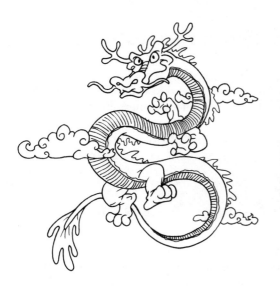

Chapter 20

Mulan Quan Basic Short Form

In This Chapter

➤ An Introduction to Mulan Quan style T'ai Chi

➤ How Mulan Quan promotes grace, beauty, and health

➤ Mulan Quan can be very good for your heart

If Mulan Quan's main benefit could be put into two words, they would be "self esteem." The artistry of its forms and the mental healing of its practice expand and enhance our self-perception. Mulan's elegant promotion of grace and agility make it perfect for women, yet great for men, too.

Mulan Quan is a rather modern form of T'ai Chi, but it is derived from an ancient, nearly extinct form of Hua Chia Quan (*Hua* is flower, *Chia* is frame, *Quan* is fist, meaning "beautiful boxing style"). The Mulan Quan T'ai Chi short form comprises 24 powerful, yet delicate movements that flow one into the other. Below is an introduction into the first 12 movements of the Mulan style of T'ai Chi. To learn the rest of this beautiful style and to supplement the information in this chapter, the video *Mulan Quan Basic Short Form*, listed in the back of this book, may be very helpful. Again, it is difficult to convey in still photographs the multidimensionality of T'ai Chi's flowing motions.

Mulan Quan Promotes Elegance

The physical elegance of Mulan Quan gives the practitioner a regal appearance that is mesmerizing. The practice of its forms has a wonderful impact on the self-esteem of its practitioners. However, the mental healing is just the beginning because this vehicle enhances our physical beauty, as well as our physical health.

Mulan Beauty Treatment

Mulan Quan is a highly effective beauty regimen for women. Its ability to simultaneously instill a sense of deep personal power and elegance in motion literally changes the practitioner's personality and outlook on life. This living embodiment of power, grace, and artistry actually transforms the practitioner. No external cosmetic can come close to the beauty treatment Mulan Quan offers. However, with a more beautiful being within, anything you adorn yourself with externally will be very effective.

Mulan the Healer

Mulan Quan is recommended for many ailments, including lower back problems, obesity, heart diseases, insomnia, and other chronic diseases. Reports from Chinese hospitals indicate Mulan Quan has been very useful in stroke rehabilitation treatment and as an adjunct therapy for cancer patients. The Beijing Cancer Center used Mulan as a physical therapy for patients, who then saw improved appetites, weight gain, and better overall health.

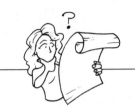

Know Your Chinese

Mulan Quan translated literally is "wooden orchid fist," which means "strong, beautiful, fist." *Mu* is wood, *lan* is orchid, and *quan* (chuan) is fist. This style is named after the brave young woman, Mulan Fa, who selflessly took her aging father's place in the war to save his life. Her story was made famous by Disney's epic animated feature, *Mulan*.

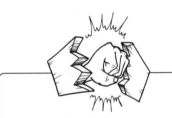

A T'ai Chi Punch Line

Chinese T'ai Chi masters often say, "You are as young as your spine is flexible."

Step East to Lotus

This series of movements rotates both upper and lower body joints, while promoting a deep sense of tranquility. These movements improve your balance and promote an expressive attitude of elegance.

Step in the Eastern Direction

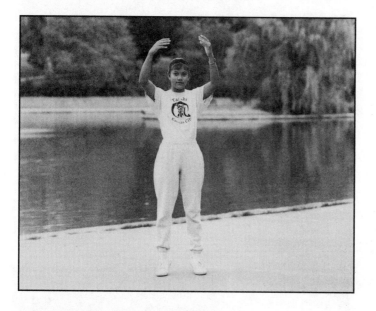

Stepping in the Eastern Direction helps you relax into your forms. This initial motion's liquid quality places the mind in a pool of tranquility as it prepares the body for what's to come.

Spread Wings on Lotus

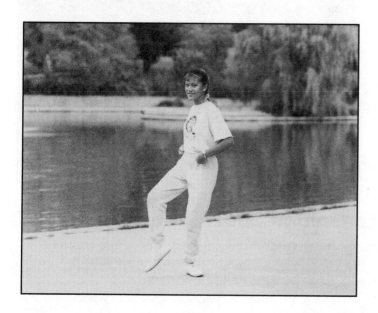

This motion fully rotates the shoulder joints, which can begin to loosen some of the daily stress we tend to accumulate there. This movement challenges and improves your ability to balance, as it carries you through a transitional move toward the next movement.

This is the preparatory movement leading to lifting the left leg.

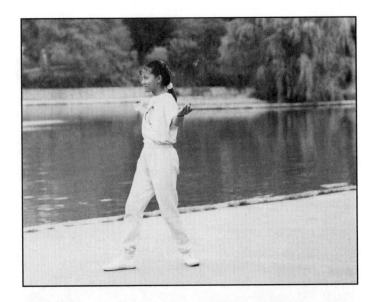

Elegance and balance are the hallmarks of this form. This movement rotates and begins to release deep tensions in the hip sockets and surrounding tissue.

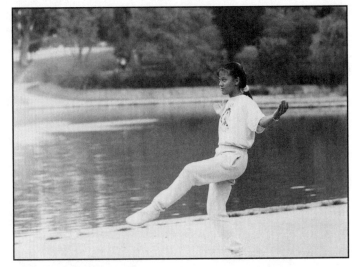

Float Rainbow to Golden Lotus

This series begins with deep loosening throughout the upper body and out to the fingers. Yet it continues to open Qi's flow throughout the entire lower body as well.

Floating Rainbow

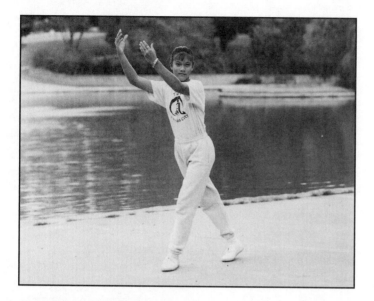

This beautiful extension lives up to its lovely name. Floating Rainbow tones the body and exercises the shoulder, elbow, wrist, and finger joints.

Sit on Golden Lotus

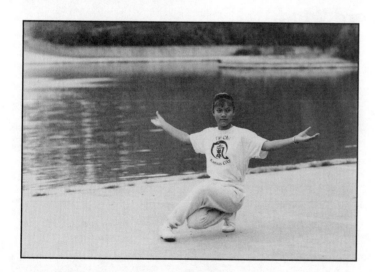

While promoting grace and balance, Sit on Golden Lotus works the thighs and legs. Some feel that the demands T'ai Chi puts on the thighs very effectively promotes circulation to the lower extremities, which allows the heart to work less hard to oxygenate the body.

Ride Wind to Dragon Flying

These motions promote a very subtle internal awareness of balance and movement. Every part of the body is worked and loosened in this series.

Ride with Wind and Waves

A very subtle shifting of the weight between the front and back legs exercises all the muscle groups in the lower body. The arm movements likewise loosen joints and tonify muscles throughout the upper body.

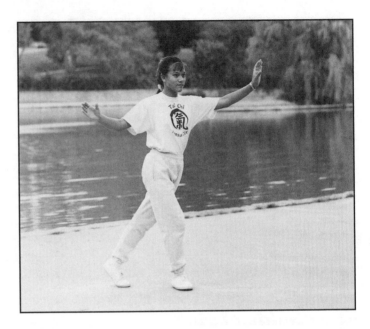

Dragon Flying Toward Wind

This movement is a very subtle internal motion that focuses awareness within.

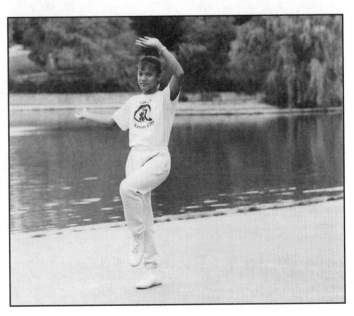

Purple Swan Tilts Its Wings

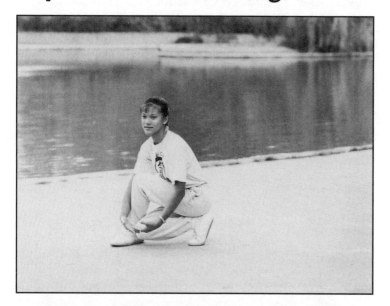

Nearly every muscle is loosened and strengthened by this move, but the abdominal muscles benefit especially. This series promotes spinal flexibility.

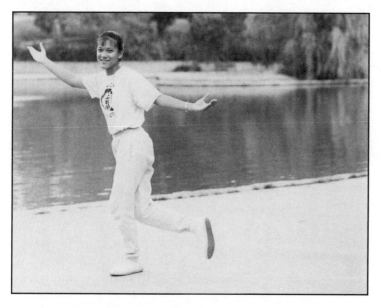

This exquisite movement is not only beautiful to the external eye but also promotes health, balance, and flexibility through the torso and spine.

The Least You Need to Know

➤ Mulan Quan movements promote elegance and balance.

➤ Mulan Quan promotes flexibility through the spine and extremities, which may keep you feeling young.

➤ Mulan Quan can tone muscles and especially strengthen the thighs, which may be very good news for your heart.

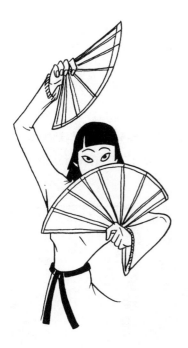

Chapter 21

Mulan Quan Fan Style

In This Chapter

➤ How T'ai Chi promotes self-esteem

➤ Mulan Quan works the entire frame

➤ Using Mulan Quan as an emotional therapy

➤ Finding the pearl within you through Mulan Quan

Mulan Quan is based in traditional T'ai Chi movement and *wushu*. However, it adds aspects of Chinese folk dance and gymnastics to provide a vessel of motion for the beauty of the practitioner to be poured into. Mulan Quan therefore reaches to the outward limits the practitioner can express, both with the wushu aspects and even as a spectacular sword form (see Chapter 22). Yet, it also explores the softest, most delicate aspects of the user, which is most beautifully expressed in the Mulan Quan fan style.

There are two fan styles, the single fan and the double fan. This chapter will introduce you to the basic single fan style. For further instruction, see the video *Mulan Quan Fan Style* listed in the back of the book. This chapter will expose you to how the forms look and will elaborate on how they are performed and what benefits each provides. But again, the motion and multidimensional quality is best learned in a live class or at least with video instruction.

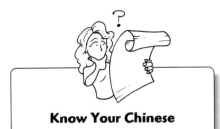

Know Your Chinese

Wushu means martial arts.

Mulan Quan styles are rapidly gaining popularity and have been involved in exhibitions and competitions from Beijing to Kansas City. Work is being done to eventually introduce Mulan Quan to Olympic competition.

Flying Bees Through Leaves

This section's movement works and stretches the entire body.

Notice here how this motion exercises the arm muscles and loosens the joints as you relax into the pose.

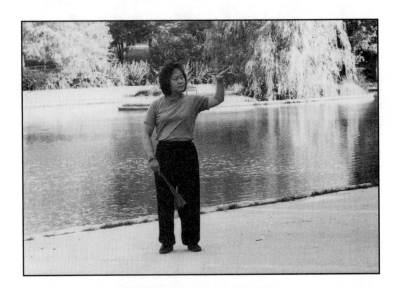

Flying Bees Through Leaves is quite graceful, but the movement is only a vessel through which to express yourself. Enjoy as you experience your own grace being poured into the vessel of your T'ai Chi. Furthermore, it tonifies the entire body from head to toe.

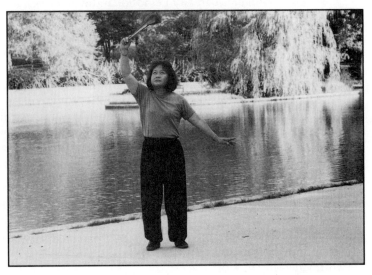

Stretching Cloud to Floating

Promoting equilibrium and refinement, this series is internal and subtle, and yet externally strengthening to all muscles.

Stretching Left Foot

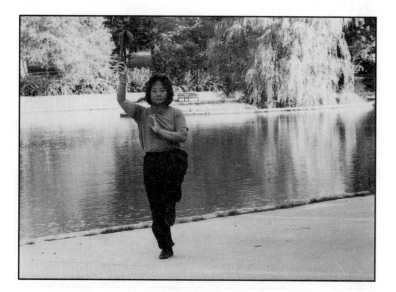

While strengthening the leg muscles, this movement fosters an internal awareness that improves your balance.

Cloud Lotus Floating

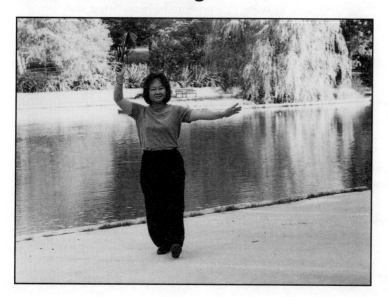

The external motion is refined by encouraging the practitioner to "feel elegant." Of course, besides that mental and spiritual benefit, it has a very practical purpose of working and loosening the arm's joints.

Miracle Touching Ocean

The beautiful names of this section are inspiring, but the movements hold even more. While creating very solid strengthening, these movements also affect the way we feel about ourselves. Mulan Quan can literally transform one's self-esteem.

Miracle Dragon Lifting Head

The Miracle Dragon Lifting Head encourages the practitioner to lengthen, enhancing and promoting good posture.

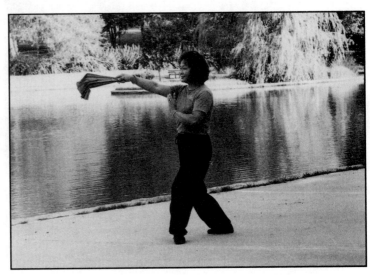

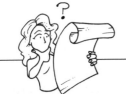

Know Your Chinese

In Chinese folklore, the **dragon** represents the *yang* (expressive) aspect of power and majesty, which may be why it is commonly used in T'ai Chi imagery to help practitioners access and evoke the limitless power of their dynamic nature.

Miracle Dragon Lifting Head is actually well-named because moving in a posture of head-lifted self-esteem (which T'ai Chi requires) actually transforms the practitioner over time in ways which may seem miraculous. Mulan Quan may be a powerful adjunct therapy for the many emotionally affected conditions, such as eating disorders, facing some young women today.

Swallow Touching Ocean

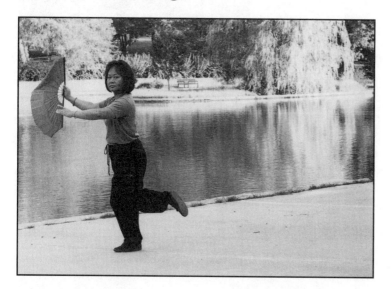

This movement powerfully strengthens the leg and back muscles, while promoting release of tension through the back.

Green Willow Twigs Dancing

This section offers great overall toning exercises, and its delicate foot work especially focuses toning in the leg.

Green Willow Twigs Swaying

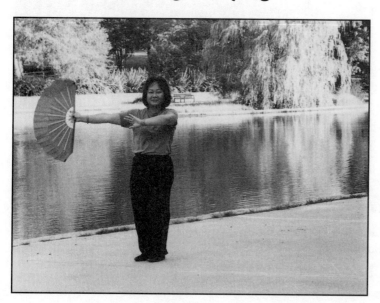

The deep rotation of the hip of Green Willow Twigs Swaying allows a subtle internal awareness of how the body shifts from its power point, or dan tien.

This posture works all the joints and muscles, offering great strengthening and toning throughout the entire frame.

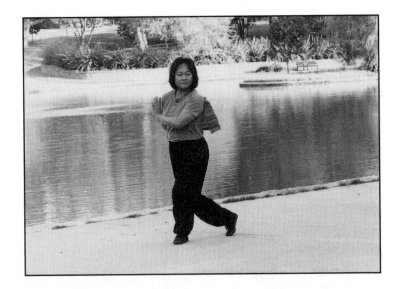

Dancing in Wind

The delicate footwork of Dancing in Wind is a great toning exercise for the legs, and its subtlety offers a meditative quality as it's performed.

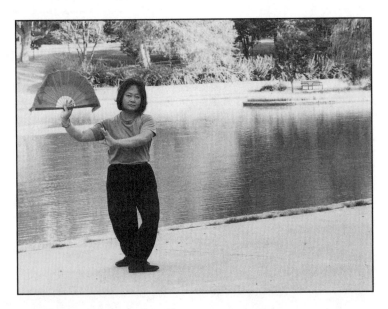

Dun Huang Flying Dance

While challenging the lower body to maintain balance, the upper body is rotated and flexed in a soothing relaxed way.

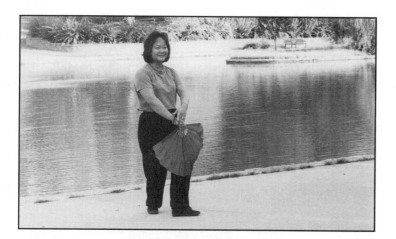

The shoulder and wrist rotations of this motion release stress and soothe the practitioner's mind as she flows through its graceful ways.

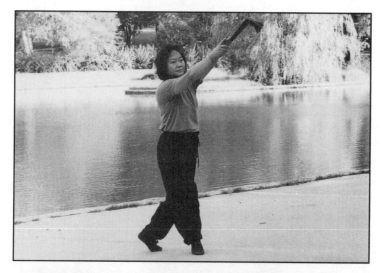

The spine and waist are flexed gently, promoting a litheness that is not only lovely but enhances all aspects of health, according to Traditional Chinese Medicine.

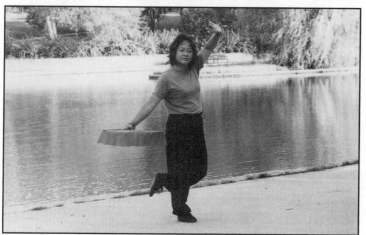

While the legs work and adjust to subtle posture changes, the upper body is gently stretched and loosened.

The Least You Need to Know

➤ Mulan Quan can change your self-image, which can positively change your physical appearance over time.

➤ Mulan Quan's self-esteem promotion may be a wonderful adjunct therapy to women facing emotional problems.

➤ The elegance Mulan Quan offers is really within you right now! Mulan Quan only helps you to express that part of yourself.

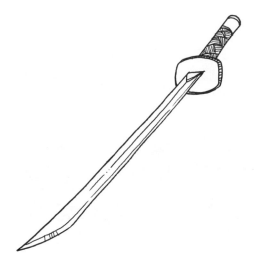

Chapter 22

Mulan Sword Form: A T'ai Chi Cut Up!

In This Chapter

➤ The sword form promotes internal power

➤ How elegance promotes balance and strength

➤ Balancing raw power and subtle beauty within your mind, heart and body

Mulan Quan is great for everyone, but again, women greatly benefit from the elegance and tender beauty it promotes. However, another profound benefit is its tremendous, yet subtle, power. The power of Mulan Quan is perhaps most dramatically observed in the performance of Mulan Quan Sword Style.

This chapter will expose you to some of the sword form postures, their benefits, and points to enrich your experience with them. It is recommended, however, that you use this book as a supplement to live classes or at least video instruction. The complexity of these lovely forms can better be comprehended when you can move, follow, and hear instructions at the same time.

Preparation to Eye on Sword

This section quietly prepares the mind and body before launching into the expansive motion of the Mulan Quan Sword Style.

Preparation Stance

The Preparation Stance is
meant to focus and relax
the mind, body, and heart.

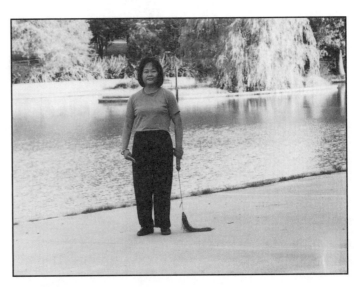

Left Foot Half Step with Eyes on Sword

Here is a full rotation of
the shoulder and arm as
the sword arm goes into a
clockwise rotation.

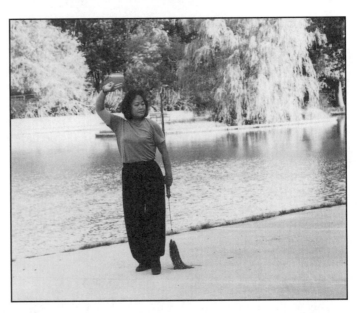

Forward Step to Low Jab

This series works the entire body, loosening and lengthening from head to toe.

Forward Step, Holding Sword Under Elbow

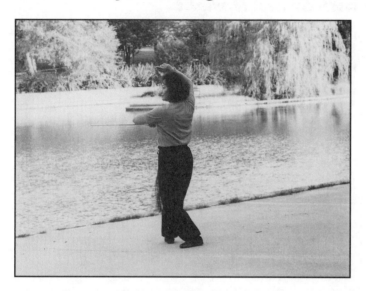

Your right foot steps right with weight shifting forward. Bring your sword-wielding arm straight out to the side, then around to the front and bent elbow. This movement helps to loosen the entire body as you breathe and allow your Qi to flow through all limbs, as well as through the sword hand.

Sword Exchange, Turn Body and Low Jab

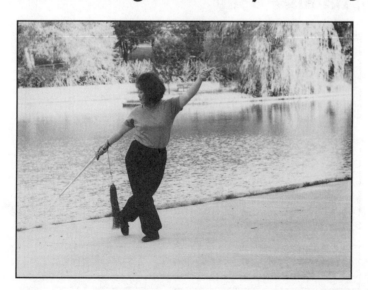

This movement fosters an elongation of the entire frame as the hips are rotated and the body loosens.

Sword Upright to Balance Body

In these motions, your entire body is strengthened with very desirable and select muscle toning.

Body Return, Step with Sword Upright

The abdominal muscles are toned in this movement as the back and legs are worked, as well.

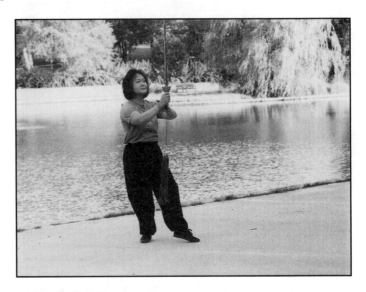

Vertical Sword and Balance Body

The shoulder and wrist joints are exercised here, which helps the practitioner avoid calcium deposit buildup in joints that might negatively affect flexibility. Mulan Quan enables us to age while maintaining fluid, elegant flexibility.

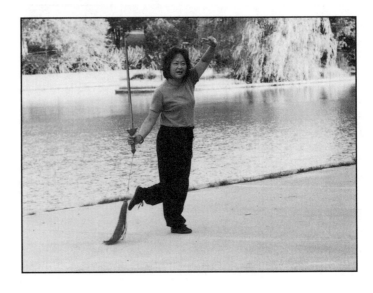

Turn Around to Up Jab

Balance, posture, and leg strength are found in this set of movements.

Turn Around, Lower to Sitting Position, Sword Upright

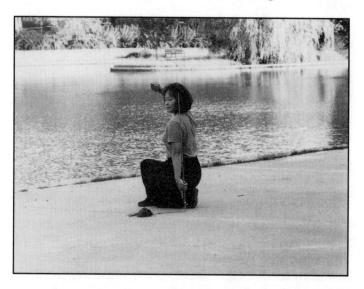

Leg muscles are both stretched and strengthened as you breathe and lengthen through this movement.

Step Up, Lower to Sitting Position, Sword Up Jab

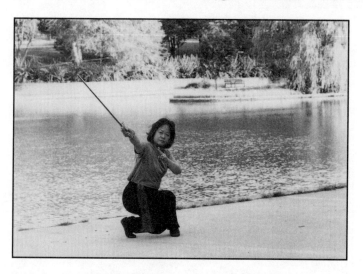

Practicing this movement with an attitude of "elegance and style" will have a wonderful impact on both your balance and your posture.

269

Level Sword to Lift Leg

The following set tonifies and beautifies in many ways.

Level Sword, Turn Body and Lift Knee

While improving your balance, Level Sword, Turn Body also tones and strengthens.

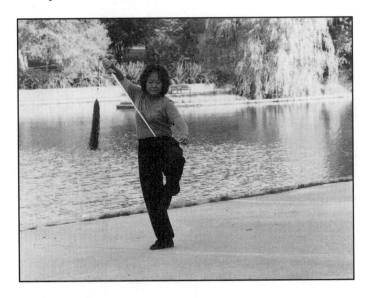

Lift Leg, Side Step, Side Chop with Sword

This may be the most beautiful of all Mulan Quan movements, yet it also works to loosen the body's muscles and joints.

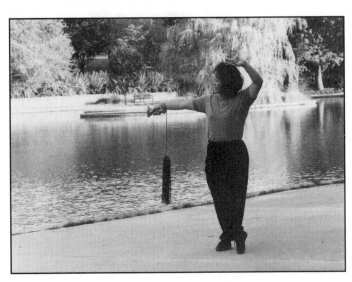

The Least You Need to Know

➤ The sword form promotes a sense of gentle power.

➤ Remember to make the forms fit your body.

➤ Let the thought of elegance elongate your form through the practice of these movements.

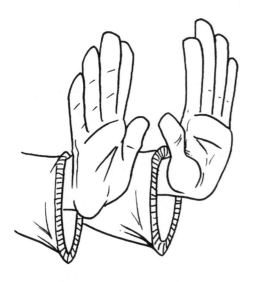

Chapter 23

Getting Gently Pushy with Push Hands

In This Chapter

➤ Learn the art of Push Hands

➤ Use Push Hands to learn about yourself

➤ How masters resist many opponents effortlessly

What Is Push Hands?

Push Hands is a paradox. It is a sparring technique in a way, but it is also a quiet tool of self-awareness. The way you see Push Hands says as much about you as it does about Push Hands. To one person it may look like a delicate dance, while another may see a physical contest not unlike a sumo-wrestling match. Actually it is a tiny bit of both.

By moving your dan tien in towards your opponent, your weight shifts toward your front foot, and your Qi flows through the body exerting a very relaxed force (like the unbendable arm). So as your hand pushes toward your opponent, if the opponent is stiff, this will likely uproot their stance, causing them to loose their balance. If they are supple and yielding, they will absorb your attack and respond in kind.

The goal, however, is not to forcefully uproot your opponent. Instead, the purpose of Push Hands is to become accustomed to the ebb and flow of physical energy expressed in motion. If your opponent is pushy and abrupt, they will likely overextend them-selves as they attack. This attack isn't violent; it's just their arm extending into your chest or heart area. When they overextend, they will come in off balance if you yield. When they retreat to try to catch their balance, they are vulnerable. A slight push can send a larger, more powerful opponent reeling when they are out of center.

When pushing hands we seek to maintain a delicate contact with our opponent, while remaining flexible and calmly aware ourselves. Push Hands is mainly about observing and responding with the most power and least effort.

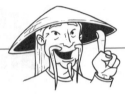

Sage Sifu Says

When pushing hands, envision a butterfly poised between your wrist and the wrist of your opponent. Try to have just enough pressure between them so the butterfly doesn't fly away, yet not so much that you crush it. Your goal is to maintain subtle contact, yielding when attacked, and advancing when the opponent yields.

Notice that the pusher is focusing his energy toward the other by facing his palm toward the opponent as he pushes. The energy center, Lao Gong, on the Pericardium energy meridian is in the center of the palm of the hand. This is a highly sensitive point and also projects energy outward.

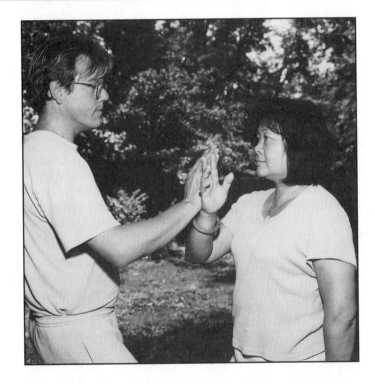

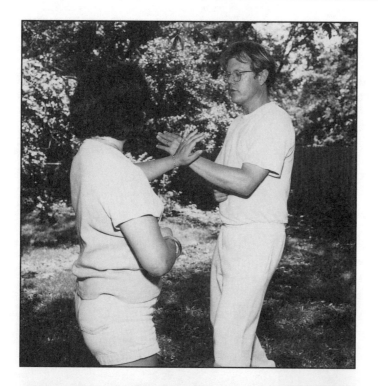

The goal of Push Hands is not to resist but to yield and deflect incoming power.

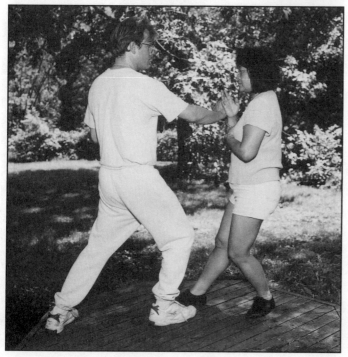

Remember the story of the snake yielding to the white crane's attacks.

Think of a butterfly resting between the exchanging hands or wrists as you push or retreat from your opponent. Try to be sensitive enough to anticipate motions so that your advancing opponent does not crush the butterfly as you lithely retreat.

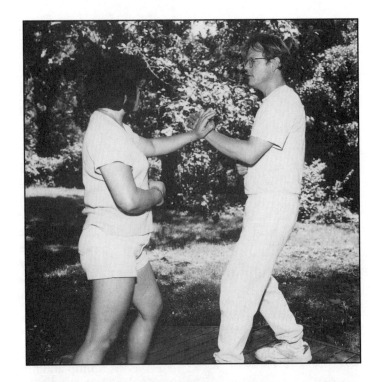

Realize that just as with all T'ai Chi, Push Hands is not physical force as we usually think of it.

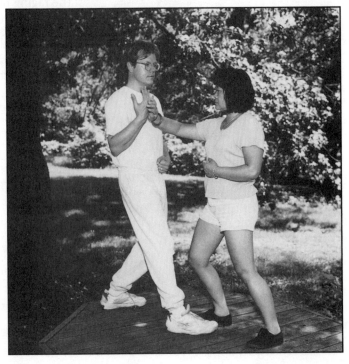

Push Hands is done with the same effortless power as the Unbendable Arm presented in Chapter 4. Also, notice that in this exercise, the unused hand is a fist held at the ready near the chest. In T'ai Chi, as in all martial arts, nothing is done without reason. The resting hand is ever ready to spring into action. We don't think in fear, but in relaxed alertness.

The Psychology of Push Hands

Again, Push Hands is about observing. As with all T'ai Chi, it is all-encompassing and has as much to teach us about our mind and heart as it does about our physical balance and dexterity.

If I am pushy and overpowering in life, this will show up in my Push Hands technique. I will often find myself overextending or overempha-

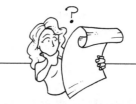

Know Your Chinese

The Chinese word **song** is used constantly in T'ai Chi. Its literal translation is "relaxation," although this doesn't quite reflect its meaning. We usually think of relaxation as flaccid limpness, but the word song reflects a relaxed power, calm but ready, soothed yet alert. The unbendable arm exercise in Chapter 4 illustrates this.

sizing the attack with little thought of staying centered. Likewise, if I am too timid, the dancing exchange of Push Hands will seem limp and lifeless—not much fun. The goal, as always, is to strike balance between both the raging bull and the shrinking violet that reside within us. Both aspects of self are perfect and absolutely necessary to making us a whole being, just as nature is perfect because it contains these extremes and everything in between.

Practicing Push Hands can raise the raging bull from the shrinking violet and bloom delicate petals from the raging bull. As T'ai Chi expands your beingness, Push Hands can help by illustrating in an external social element the internal tendencies you may not have noticed about yourself or others.

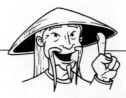

Sage Sifu Says

The expanded awareness and practice of experiencing different aspects of self that Push Hands promotes makes us more fluid and better able to become whatever is required and most useful at any given moment. Push Hands is training in being all things.

Eventually, Push Hands may become a powerful business or marriage-counseling tool because it helps to illuminate how people interact. Its not about labeling one person's technique as good or bad, but rather about becoming aware of people's tendencies so that we can interact more effectively no matter where they are coming from.

Different Forms of Push Hands

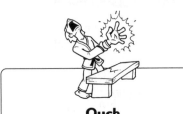

Ouch

For those in a more frail physical condition using T'ai Chi as therapy, more martial Push Hands techniques are ill advised and really not necessary you can play with a basic Push Hands routine with a partner you can trust to be gentle enough. Or you can skip Push Hands all together. As always, these tools are toys to play with. We only play with toys we enjoy and make us feel good, which is the point of toys in the first place.

There are several different forms of Push Hands. Some incorporate very directly applicable martial techniques that involve deflecting blows and tripping your opponent as they loose their balance. These are fun, but not necessary for most T'ai Chi training. If you are curious about these techniques, shop around for an instructor well versed in Push Hands. If your instructor does not do Push Hands, you may find weekend workshops that teach the techniques, or perhaps there may be someone who knows at T'ai Chi club gatherings. Contacting the T'ai Chi organizations listed in the back of this book may help lead you to teachers or events that specialize in push hands.

It's playtime.

Legends of the Masters

There are stories about T'ai Chi masters who exhibit almost superhuman strength when being pushed or when pushing others. Bill Moyer's documentary on the healing mind showed an old Chinese master that could withstand the onslaught of a half dozen pushing students without being budged and seemingly without really exerting himself. This same master also sent those students flying off across the lawn with hardly any indication of movement on his part.

There is an area of T'ai Chi that focuses on energy projection called "fa-jing", and it is claimed that some masters (like the one Bill Moyer met) can use the force of their Qi to withstand attacks and send opponents flying. However, there may be a physical element to this ability as well.

If the human body is a structure like a building, then engineering principles may explain some of this. If just the right structuring of materials in just the right way can build buildings that resist massive pressure in weight-bearing demands, can't the body likewise do so? If a T'ai Chi master were very attuned to how his body aligned bones and muscles with the support of the earth beneath, he may be able to resist great external force by using internal engineering principles. Also, as in Push Hands, if one was so self-aware of these principles, one could be subtly attuned to when this opponent offered the slightest break in their solidity. Then, the master would be able to uproot the opponents with the least bit of force. This would seem magical to the untrained eye, just as a remote control would seem magical to a cave man. However, it may really be just a matter of subtle awareness.

The Least You Need to Know

➤ Push Hands helps you become self-aware.

➤ Push Hands improves balance and power.

➤ For those rehabilitating from injuries or with balance problems, Push Hands may best be avoided.

Part 6
Life Applications

Part 6 will show how T'ai Chi can change your life and our world. T'ai Chi becomes a gateway to looking at life and health in a completely different way. By seeing our world and ourselves in a proactively empowered way, we can literally change the course of our lives and make our world a much better place.

Part 6 will detail illnesses T'ai Chi can help treat and how corporations can support their employees development of healthy lifestyles, while maximizing profits by increasing productivity. T'ai Chi's power to reduce stress and positively treat nearly any illness can improve the bottom line profits of any corporation. This is why T'ai Chi is becoming the single most powerful step we can take to resolve our health crisis and economic woes. Eighty percent of illness is due to stress, and U.S. businesses are losing $300 billion per year ($7,500 per employee per year) due to stress-related problems.

It seems there is literally no physical or social problem that cannot be powerfully treated with the calming healing balm T'ai Chi and QiGong offer our harried world. So, Part 6 will offer some suggestions and present some examples of how others have introduced T'ai Chi into their workplace, schools, hospitals, and communities.

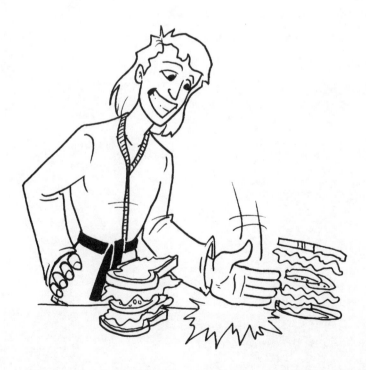

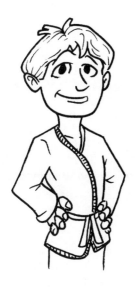

Chapter 24

T'ai Chi for Special People and as Therapy

In This Chapter

➤ T'ai Chi is great for kids, if taught correctly

➤ T'ai Chi saves senior's lives

➤ Women find T'ai Chi powerful therapy

➤ T'ai Chi helps men develop their softer side

➤ Get the edge in sports using T'ai Chi

➤ T'ai Chi is a great healing therapy

T'ai Chi is for everyone. This chapter will provide details on how T'ai Chi benefits specific people, their health conditions, and their athletic activities.

If you are treating a specific condition, you will find an introduction to how T'ai Chi may assist your ongoing therapy. For seniors, you will find out why T'ai Chi is the very best thing you can do for yourself. Specific reasons why children, men, and women should practice T'ai Chi are provided as well.

This chapter will also assist parents and/or T'ai Chi teachers who want to start a T'ai Chi class for kids. Kids are taught differently from adults, and this chapter will give teachers or parents some great insights into helping their kids make the most of T'ai Chi, and have fun doing it.

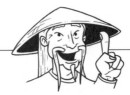

Sage Sifu Says

There are many T'ai Chi classes and teachers. Find the one right for you.

T'ai Chi for Kids

Kids are the embodiment of change, and change can be very stressful. Their minds and bodies grow at phenomenal rates, so they are constantly having to work with new and different bodies, making coordination and balance a big issue. T'ai Chi, with its emphasis on balance, is well suited to address all of these challenges.

Athletic Improvement for Kids

T'ai Chi works to integrate the mind and body, skeletal and muscular systems, and left brain and right brain. In physical terms, this centering is built around an awareness of moving with good posture and from a low center of gravity, or the vertical axis and the dan tien.

Gifted athletes are people who are naturals at this kind of self-awareness and movement. Since most of our kids are not naturals, T'ai Chi can be a most effective way to help your child prepare for athletics and to simply be comfortable in their rapidly changing bodies.

Ouch!

Check with your child's therapist or physician before beginning T'ai Chi. Also, find an effective, understanding T'ai Chi instructor who has experience teaching children.

Attention Deficit Disorder (ADD)

ADD is a growing problem not only with children, but adults as well. T'ai Chi may be a wonderful adjunct therapy for treating ADD because it augments many of the mood management techniques recommended for ADD sufferers.

Drs. Edward M. Hallowell, M.D., and John J. Ratey, M.D., experts on the management of ADD wrote, "Exercise is positively one of the best treatments for ADD. It helps work off excess energy and aggression in a positive way, it allows for noise-reduction within the mind, it stimulates the hormonal and neurochemical system in a most therapeutic way, and it soothes and calms the body."

The slow mindful movements of T'ai Chi have much to offer people who suffer from ADD. The following table explains why T'ai Chi may be a perfect ADD therapy:

T'ai Chi and ADD

What Experts Suggest	What T'ai Chi Offers
Set aside time for recharging batteries, something calm and restful, like meditation	T'ai Chi is a mini-vacation
Daily exercise that is readily available and needs little preparation can help with the blahs that occur and with overall outlook	T'ai Chi is easy, requires no preparation, and is a daily mood elevator
Observe mood swings; learn to accept them by realizing they will pass. Learn strategies that might help bad moods pass sooner.	T'ai Chi is a tool for self-observation of feelings and for letting those feelings go
Use "time-outs" when you are upset or over-stimulated; take a time-out; go away, calm down	T'ai Chi can be performed in the bathroom at school or work, giving you a break from the stress
Let go of the urgency to always finish things quickly by learning to enjoy the process	T'ai Chi's slow flowing routine is about letting go of outcome and learning to love process
ADD usually includes a tendency to overfocus or hyperfocus at times, to obsess or ruminate over some imagined problem without being able to let it go	T'ai Chi teaches the practice of letting go on a mental, emotional, and physical level with each exhale

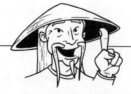

Sage Sifu Says

Realize that T'ai Chi for kids with ADD will not look like T'ai Chi for adults. It will be faster. See the section on teaching kids.

How Do You Teach T'ai Chi to Kids?

Not just kids with A.D.D., but all kids usually have difficulty with the slowness of T'ai Chi. Therefore, you simply speed it up. Teach each child at their own pace; some can go slower than others can.

Give kids constant recognition for their T'ai Chi accomplishments. Ask each kid to demonstrate his or her new movements for the class at the end and have everyone applaud. If a kid forgets a move, jump in and do it with them. Over the weeks, they will look forward to the recognition and practice more.

T'ai Chi is a loose thing, not a rigid thing. It can work for everybody and can be taught in many fun ways. Keep a kid's T'ai Chi class moving and include stretching exercises from yoga or aggressive calisthenics to use up excess energy. Then, as the kids get more tired, you can ease them into slower movement.

Kids can do QiGong meditations, too. It isn't anything like adult meditations; there are more and different images that work. Try the children's meditation tape offered in the back of this book for examples.

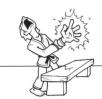

Ouch!

Each condition is different, so check with your physician to discuss T'ai Chi's potential benefits to your case. T'ai Chi is extremely gentle and should not be confused with the harder martial arts, but consult your doctor before beginning class.

T'ai Chi for Seniors

Seniors can find no better exercise in the world than T'ai Chi. T'ai Chi may help build bone mass and connective tissue, with zero joint damage, according to some studies. Other studies show that T'ai Chi is twice as good as any other balance exercise in the world. Since complications from falling injuries are the sixth largest cause of death among seniors, this is a very big deal. For seniors with chronic conditions, there are many maladies that T'ai Chi can help treat. These are listed later in this chapter.

If your mobility is limited in some way, that is no problem, even if you're in a wheelchair. There is a class for you, and if you are persistent, you'll find a teacher and a class that are perfect.

T'ai Chi for Women

There are many reasons why T'ai Chi is the ultimate exercise for women. Its ability to cultivate both elegance and power are two of these. In today's working environment where women are competing in the workforce with men and trying to break through the glass ceiling, T'ai Chi's ability to cultivate an inner sense of confident power can be very helpful. However, there are many biological reasons T'ai Chi can be helpful to women as well.

Bone Loss

Bone loss is a big problem with many women. Studies indicate that stress may be a major factor contributing to the loss of bone mass in even relatively young women. The daily stress release T'ai Chi promotes provides a powerful preventative therapy to help ensure a long active life for women.

For women including those over 45, studies have shown that QiGong practice raises estrogen levels. This is highly desirable because reduced estrogen levels after menopause cause a loss of calcium from the bones and increase the risk of osteoporosis and heart disease.

Eating Disorders

Women suffer from eating disorders ten times as often as men. Although often thought of as an adult problem, anorexia and bulimia most often start in the teenage years while the sufferer is still at home. Although I am unaware of any studies on the effectiveness of T'ai Chi as therapy for anorexia or bulimia, the underlying issues and symptomology seem to suggest that much of the treatment criteria are embodied in T'ai Chi practice.

For example, it is recommended that anorexia or bulimia sufferers strengthen their inner core of self and self-worth. The self-esteem that T'ai Chi practice builds and encourages can be a highly effective way to discover the power within one's self. The need for a restoration of biochemical and hormonal balance may be facilitated with T'ai

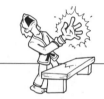

Ouch!

As always, do not attempt to self-treat any disorder, including an eating disorder. Suggest T'ai Chi and QiGong to your physician or therapist as an adjunct therapy. It may be a powerful addition to your ongoing treatment, but discuss it with your doctor.

Chi's ability to create a homeostatic effect throughout the body, not only physically, but also mentally and emotionally. T'ai Chi addresses the need to balance internal rhythms and needs with life's demands by those who practice it so they can become quietly mindful of subtle feelings and needs before they become a crisis born out in acute stress or panic.

Mood swings and depression are a part of bulimic bingeing, and feelings of lack of personal control are a part of many teenagers' anorexia or bulimia. Food, or denying ourselves food, provides us with a feeling of self-control over a world out of control. T'ai Chi's regular practice is designed to help us realize that we have a great deal of control over how we are impacted by the world. This centering enables us to feel more accepting of the fact that much of the world is beyond our control.

Pregnancy

T'ai Chi has much to offer a pregnant woman, if practiced very gently and with care. It is a slow and gentle exercise that can be performed by most pregnant women. Its gentleness and relaxed motion promotes the circulation of energy and blood throughout the body, while its smooth abdominal breathing fully oxygenates the body of both mother and child. However, *only practice when it feels good* and *never strain yourself*. Rest whenever you need to and modify or forego any movement or exercise that doesn't feel right.

T'ai Chi breathing is a wonderful way to prepare for delivery. The famous Lamaze Technique is based on QiGong breathing techniques and pain management tools. This aspect of T'ai Chi makes it perhaps the most effective exercise to prepare you for a safe natural childbirth. Remember to breathe.

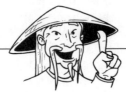

Sage Sifu Says

For pregnant women, although T'ai Chi is very gentle, some postures may be too low or somewhat strenuous. Do not practice these or adjust them so they are less strenuous. As your pregnancy progresses, change your T'ai Chi to make it less strenuous with each passing month. Always go slow and listen to your body. Do not do anything that doesn't feel good. Be sure your physician approves of T'ai Chi before beginning classes.

T'ai Chi for Men

Just as T'ai Chi can help women to develop their powerful dynamic side, T'ai Chi helps men develop their passive or receptive side as well, thereby helping men to become better homemakers and parents.

T'ai Chi's goal is to strike a balance between our dynamic (male/yang) side and our receptive (female/yin) side. Men and women have both qualities, and T'ai Chi helps us balance them.

T'ai Chi helps us let go of old self-concepts and prejudices, just as it teaches us to let go of tensions and fears. As our physical bodies relax and become more fluid, we become more flexible mentally and emotionally as well.

However, T'ai Chi can help you be that big strapping stud of an athlete as well. In fact, maybe it can help you keep up with the women who are today advancing in every sport.

T'ai Chi and Sports

T'ai Chi is the ultimate sports training tool because its goal is to cultivate balance, calm, and power, the basis for excelling in any physical activity. T'ai Chi can enhance any athletic performance. T'ai Chi's cultivation of awareness of the dan tien, or center of gravity, can be especially helpful for surfing, skateboarding, snow boarding and skiing. In fact, a T'ai Chi instructor named Chris Luth conducts "T'ai Chi Skiing Workshops."

T'ai Chi and Weight Training

Gil Messenger, a student of Master Kuo Lien-ying, was a sports trainer as well as a T'ai Chi instructor. He often taught a form of QiGong meditation to weight trainers, who were surprised to discover that they could then lift more weight. We think when we are pumped and straining we are more powerful, but these weight lifters discovered that by allowing the body to let go, to fill with light, and to move from a calm center, they increased their physical power.

T'ai Chi and Golf

In golf, instructors encourage you to "swing with the belly button." This is another way of saying to swing with the dan tien. Many golfers discover that they can drive the ball much farther after practicing T'ai Chi for only a few months.

Also, T'ai Chi's relaxed motion allows the limbs to be swung by the dan tien's motion with no muscle resistance. This in turn allows the entire force of the dan tien's turning to be projected outward through the hands and club into the ball.

Ouch!

The concept of swinging from the dan tien may also help reduce "golfer's back" problems. By thinking of swinging from below the navel (or dan tien) rather than from the navel, there is less twisting of the lower back.

T'ai Chi for Tennis and Racquetball

The same force used in golf is brought to bear in tennis and racquetball. If you play tennis or racquetball, you will also find an increased sense of control. Sometimes tennis players will describe a sense of slowing down, as if T'ai Chi practice made the game seem a bit slower than before.

Tennis players will also often discover less pressure in the knees after practicing T'ai Chi. Consciously moving from the dan tien can bring less pressure to bear on the knees when coming to an abrupt halt because when the head or upper body leads the movement, the knees must work harder to stop your momentum. T'ai Chi can also give you an off day exercise that is soothing to the joints, but still keeps the mind and body working together at a fine edge. You may be able to have fewer days on the court, while still improving your game, which may save your knees as well.

T'ai Chi and Baseball

The concept of swinging with the dan tien is exemplified in baseball's batting motion. Many batting coaches speak of "squashing the bug," which is another way of saying swing with the dan tien or body. An imaginary bug beneath the back foot is squashed as the body pulls the bat around and the back foot pivots. When performed correctly, the most powerful swings appear almost effortless. The mental calming and focus that T'ai Chi promotes can also improve the hit to strike ratio, as well as improving defensive reactions when fielding.

T'ai Chi's ability to improve balance is excellent for infielders, who must move on a dime and reach outward to make plays. However, pitchers are probably the greatest beneficiaries of T'ai Chi training. Just before going into a pitch, pitchers must for a moment hold their balance on one leg. This moment of balance is the most crucial point in a pitcher's windup and can determine both force and accuracy. Therefore, the amazing balance improvement T'ai Chi provides can be the most powerful weapon in a pitcher's arsenal.

T'ai Chi and the "Hard" Martial Arts

In the 1970s, the world was surprised to see a 19-year-old Canadian win the World Karate Championship. His secret was T'ai Chi. The centering, balance, looseness, and focus T'ai Chi promotes will greatly enhance the power and speed of any boxer or martial artist. More than any other exercise, T'ai Chi promotes increased reaction speed because it is therapy for not just external muscular performance, but for the mental and neural processes as well.

T'ai Chi as Therapy

Below are introductions to how and why T'ai Chi and/or QiGong may be an effective therapy for your condition. If you or your doctor are interested in more in-depth explanations, Master Ken Cohen's book, *The Way of QiGong: The Art and Science of Chinese Energy Healing*, may be very helpful (see bibliography).

Treating Cancer

In Chinese hospitals, T'ai Chi and QiGong are often used in conjunction with chemo- or radiation therapies. QiGong and T'ai Chi therapies can lessen the side effects of radiation treatments, but T'ai Chi has many other benefits to offer. For example, a sense of hopelessness or helplessness can diminish the effectiveness of standard treatments. T'ai Chi, however, engages the patient in the healing process, giving them a sense of empowerment.

In China, QiGong may be a primary therapy for advanced, inoperable, and medically untreatable cancer. It can slow the progression of the disease, while maintaining appetite and helping with pain management. Beyond that, the emotional and mental clarifying aspects of T'ai Chi and QiGong can also help a patient prepare for their life transition in a more meaningful and spiritual way. By helping them to become more at peace in their lives, they may find the transition to death a less fearful event, thereby enabling them to make the most of their remaining days.

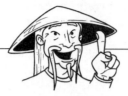

Sage Sifu Says

When you release a deep breath, think of the muscles letting go of the bones. On the next exhale, think of the brain, the mind, and the cranial muscles letting go of thoughts and worries. On the next release of breath, think of letting the heart and the muscles around it relax. Each release of breath becomes a deep cleansing and letting go on many different levels: physical, emotional, mental, and other levels we're not conscious of.

Cardiac Rehab and Prevention

Many cardiologists are prescribing T'ai Chi as an adjunct therapy for treatment of heart problems or as preventative therapy. T'ai Chi provides a gentle exercise that promotes circulation, but its meditative quality may offer even more benefits. T'ai Chi's stress reduction qualities foster a feeling of self-acceptance and safety in the world, allowing practitioners to let go of the control issues that can make life seem like an endless state of panic.

Again, T'ai Chi gives us a daily dosage of homeostatic feelings of well-being. As we become familiar with this feeling of optimum health, we get more attuned with what foods, drinks, or activities promote or detract from that wonderful feeling. This bio-feedback feature can be instrumental in helping people make lifestyle changes that may extend their lives by many years.

Stroke Recovery

Doctors now often recommend T'ai Chi for stroke recovery because T'ai Chi's soothing demands of left brain-right brain interaction and mind-body interaction can epitomize a physical therapy for stroke victims. T'ai Chi challenges patients to coordinate movement, but at the same time helps them feel at ease in the face of the frustration this challenge might cause. If balance is a severe problem, a spouse or friend can spot you to help maintain balance.

Ouch!

If you have a balance disorder and wish to use a climbing harness to prevent falls, discuss the exact purpose of the harness with a climbing expert. This will enable them to ensure the harness you use is appropriate to keep you from falling. This security will help you relax more, thereby allowing you to get more benefit from T'ai Chi. Ask the expert about the full-body harness, often used in caving as well as climbing.

In Kansas City, we are pioneering a new approach to T'ai Chi for stroke victims with balance problems. By securing a mountain climbing harness to the ceiling by a hook, a patient may perform T'ai Chi without fear of falling. One of the main balance benefits all T'ai Chi practitioners get comes from constantly testing the limits of their balance. As one drifts in and out of balance, the mind and body exchange data that effortlessly improves the balance, which often continues to improve for life. The figure below shows the harness approach. Note that the harness below is only illustrative and not sufficient to prevent falls; *a full-body harness, including a shoulder harness that secures in front of the upper chest, is required to prevent falling.*

Hospitals all over the world eventually will provide rooms filled with hooks for climbing harnesses so that stroke rehab or other balance-challenged patients can come and practice T'ai Chi without fear of falling. These same patients may wish to have harnesses installed in their homes by a qualified contractor. Contact your hospital and show them this section. Physical therapists can consult with mountain climbing supply stores to find the optimum full-body harnesses.

Do not use this harness to prevent falls.

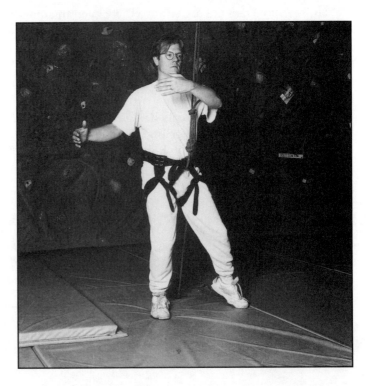

Addictions

T'ai Chi, as well as acupuncture, is being successfully used to help people break addictive patterns. Breaking an addiction, whether its to cigarettes or heroin, is a very stressful endeavor. The body and mind crave and yearn constantly.

What is it that they crave? Ultimately it is life energy. When a smoker gets a cigarette or an addict gets their fix, the first thing they do is sit back, enjoy the moment, and relax into the pleasure of their cigarette or fix. This moment of relaxed focused awareness opens their mind and body to an increased flow of Qi or energy. This is why a raging drunk can have so much energy, even when filled with alcohol. The problem is the cigarettes or drugs are destroying your body to open up to Qi, and when the drug wears off, the body clamps down, squeezing off the flow even more. So, learning to open to Qi in a healthy, expansive way is one means for healing an addiction.

Note the pattern of addiction:

1. A prospective user is looking for access to Qi, or life energy, whether they realize it or not. When Qi is flowing through us we feel good, at peace, and capable.

2. When cigarettes, drugs, or alcohol are first used, the ritual of using them and/or the chemical they put in the body causes the user to relax and open to Qi flow. But this is a false and unhealthy way to open to it.

3. Since this is an artificial way to open up to the flow of Qi, the mind and body do not learn how to keep the flow open.

4. In fact, when the drug, whether it's nicotine or heroin, is gone, the body and mind tighten up even more than before. The chemicals and their reactions in the body are unhealthy and cause the mind and body to get tighter, squeezing off more Qi than ever before.

5. The user is then required to use more of the drug or to use it more and more often because now it takes a more forceful dose to open the mind's and body's gates to allow the Qi to flow through.

6. Eventually, the user's dosages, no matter how large, do not open the user to increased Qi flow or a feeling of "highness." Eventually even the largest dosages give the user only a lower-than-normal flow of Qi.

7. People who are heavily hooked on cigarettes or alcohol, and even more so with harder drugs, have a look of lacking life. They are becoming void of Qi. Their mind and body have become tight.

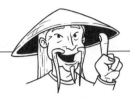

Sage Sifu Says

The more we can tap into ways to fill with life energy, using tools like T'ai Chi, the less we will have to look outside ourselves for satisfaction. Our consumption level drops as our needs diminish. Therefore, T'ai Chi can also help the environment because less consumption means less trash.

T'ai Chi and QiGong provide us with a healthy pattern of access to life energy, or Qi. This is what we all want. When we hug a loved one, we feel their Qi mingling with ours. When we pet our dog or cat, they revel in feeling our loving intention in our Qi flowing from our hand to their body. T'ai Chi and QiGong are tools to fill us with life, and they can be very effective tools for helping addicts find their way out of the maze they have stumbled into, finding a way back to being truly alive.

T'ai Chi and QiGong Are Therapeutic for Many Things

Although T'ai Chi and QiGong can play a positive role in many existing conditions, each condition is different, and you must discuss T'ai Chi as an adjunct therapy with your physician.

The following list contains some conditions T'ai Chi and/or QiGong meditations may help:

➤ **ADD.** Although the author is unaware of studies on the effectiveness of T'ai Chi as an Attention Deficit Disorder therapy, T'ai Chi meets many of the criteria for mood management techniques recommended for ADD (see beginning of chapter).

➤ **AIDS.** Studies indicate regular T'ai Chi practice may boost one's T-Cell count, while improving outlook, and providing a soothing gentle exercise. The relaxed forms effectively oxygenate the body while moving blood and lymph throughout.

➤ **Allergies and asthma.** The stress reduction benefits of T'ai Chi and QiGong help the body maintain elevated DHEA levels. Low DHEA levels have been directly linked to allergies. High stress levels are linked to the frequency and intensity of asthmatic reactions as well.

➤ **Angina.** Biofeedback aspects of T'ai Chi and QiGong can help students learn to regulate blood flow, by awareness of warmth in hands and feet. Evidence suggests this skill may alleviate some forms of angina.

➤ **Anorexia/bulimia.** See the "T'ai Chi for Women" section above.

➤ **Anxiety, chronic.** The relaxed abdominal breathing that T'ai Chi and QiGong promote can be a beneficial adjunct to therapy.

➤ **Arthritis.** T'ai Chi's low impact causes no joint damage (unlike other higher impact exercises), while its weight-bearing aspect may encourage development of bone mass and connective tissue.

➤ **Balance disorders.** T'ai Chi practitioners fall only half as much as those practicing other balance training.

➤ **Baldness, premature.** QiGong and T'ai Chi promote stress management and blood circulation. Some QiGong exercises, such as Carry the Moon, specifically promote circulation in the scalp.

➤ **Bronchitis/emphysema, chronic.** Sitting QiGong and/or T'ai Chi may show positive results over time in appetite, sleep, and energy levels, but also rather dramatically and healthfully in decreasing breaths per minute.

➤ **Pain, chronic.** Students often find anything between mild pain relief and complete alleviation of chronic pain by using T'ai Chi and/or QiGong.

➤ **Circulation and nervous system disorders.** T'ai Chi promotes circulation and can have a very integrating affect on the mind and body.

➤ **Compulsive/obsessive disorders.** T'ai Chi and QiGong's mindful awareness of self and constant reassurance that we can breathe through and relax into any situation may be a helpful adjunct to therapy for OCD, which gently exposes patients to their fears. Again, introduce T'ai Chi and QiGong only with your therapist's approval.

➤ **Depression and mood disturbance.** Regular (daily) T'ai Chi practitioners usually find less incidence of depression and overall mood disturbance.

➤ **Diabetes.** T'ai Chi's stress management and increased circulation qualities make it ideal for diabetes.

➤ **Digestion, improving.** T'ai Chi's gentle massage of internal organs, and stimulation of blood circulation and Qi promote healthy digestion.

➤ **Hemorrhoids.** Some QiGong breathing involves the sphincter muscles, which may directly alleviate hemorrhoid symptoms. T'ai Chi's ability to reduce constipation lessens the aggravation of hemorrhoid symptoms.

➤ **High blood pressure.** T'ai Chi can significantly lower high blood pressure in many cases.

T'ai Sci

Modern psychologists refer to a state of mental and emotional well-being as **homeostasis** or a homeostatic state. *T'ai Chi* promotes this by smoothing our Qi, the life blood of our mental, emotional and physical being. *T'ai Chi* is the epitome of a homeostatic exercise.

➤ **Infections.** Regular T'ai Chi practice is believed to increase the T-Cell count. T-Cells are thought to consume virus, bacteria, and even tumor cells.

➤ **Insomnia.** Students often remark of improved sleep and reduced insomnia after a few weeks of regular T'ai Chi and QiGong practice.

➤ **Lou Gehrig's disease.** T'ai Chi is recommended by many support groups of neuromuscular diseases. Check with your doctor to discuss introducing T'ai Chi as an adjunct to your therapy.

➤ **Migraine.** Biofeedback aspects of T'ai Chi and QiGong can help students learn to regulate blood flow by increasing awareness of warmth in hands and feet. Evidence suggests this skill may alleviate some forms of migraine.

➤ **Multiple sclerosis.** MS support groups recommend T'ai Chi.

➤ **Muscle wasting (and other tissue deterioration).** Studies indicate that T'ai Chi may be an ideal exercise to help older people suffering muscle wasting.

➤ **Parkinson's/improving motor-skill control.** Parkinson's support groups recommend T'ai Chi, and many students claim significant reduction in tremors.

➤ **Posture problems.** T'ai Chi's gentle mindful awareness of postural adjustment make it a wonderful therapy for posture problems and for alleviating the pain or chronic tension associated with them.

➤ **Sexual performance.** T'ai Chi's stress reduction and promotion of circulation can make it a very healthful way to improve sexual performance.

➤ **Ulcers.** QiGong relaxation therapy coupled with reductions in external stress factors have shown substantial success, even with long term ulcer problems.

➤ **Weight loss.** T'ai Chi promotes healthy weight loss in many ways. It burns calories, but also helps reduce stress levels. This stress reduction helps reduce nervous snacking. Furthermore, T'ai Chi's slow quiet mindfulness also helps us to get in touch with our *homeostatic* or healthful potential, and what that feels like. This steers us away from foods or activities that do not promote health and toward those that do.

The Least You Need to Know

➤ T'ai Chi helps kids with physical development and focus.

➤ Teach kids faster T'ai Chi and spice it up with harder exercises.

➤ T'ai Chi is perfect for kids, seniors, women, men, and athletes for many different reasons.

➤ If your physician or therapist is unfamiliar with T'ai Chi and QiGong, show them this book.

➤ No matter what ailment you have, T'ai Chi and/or QiGong can probably help.

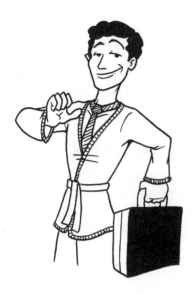

Chapter 25

"Tie"-Chi: Corporate T'ai Chi

In This Chapter

➤ How starting a T'ai Chi program at work can support your own personal T'ai Chi practice

➤ How T'ai Chi can mean big bottom-line savings

➤ Which corporations are using T'ai Chi

➤ T'ai Chi may reduce Repetitive Stress Injury

➤ T'ai Chi can enhance creativity and productivity

➤ Ways to incorporate T'ai Chi into your office or workplace

Corporations all over America are integrating the powerful health and personal growth tools of T'ai Chi into the fabric of the workplace. Why? Because T'ai Chi can save companies big money, is very applicable to the office, can lessen workplace injury, reduce stress, and boost performance.

This chapter will detail how T'ai Chi accomplishes these goals, so that you can speak with authority to your company's Wellness Director about it. Many companies will pay for a T'ai Chi program, making it well worth your time to suggest it to the Wellness Director.

A growing selection of T'ai Chi programs are now being offered in many cities by T'ai Chi, stress management, or wellness program consulting companies. To get more information on organizations or companies that offer them, check the World Wide Web or Yellow Pages under the above mentioned headings. Also, contact information is provided in the back of the book for Stress Management and Relaxation Technology (SMART) which offers such programs.

The Bottom Line on Stress Costs to Business

You can help your company understand how sponsoring T'ai Chi classes is in their best interest as well as yours. One of corporate America's highest unnecessary production costs is in lost productivity *due to employee stress*. U.S. business is losing $300 billion per year due to stress (that's over $7,500 per employee, per year), which may be why the Occupational Safety and Hazard Administration (OSHA) has declared stress a workplace hazard.

Who Is Using T'ai Chi

Companies and corporations are increasingly turning to T'ai Chi as a solution to stress. A few companies that have offered T'ai Chi to either their employees, clients, or executive staffs have been Sprint, Hallmark, Inc., Black & Veatch Corp., Associated Wholesale Grocers, BMA (Financial), and Columbia Hospitals, to name a few.

Penthouse T'ai Chi at BMA's Headquarters has been a popular wellness program. Approximately 100 employees attended the introductory Stress Management workshop.

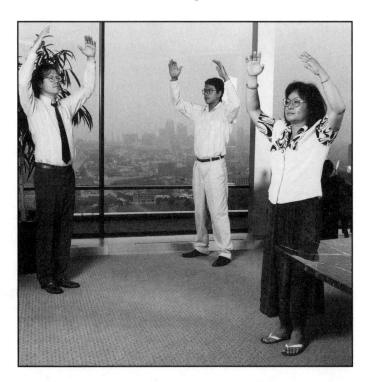

Investing in Creative Potential

If T'ai Chi can help employees recover from illnesses and thereby reduce absenteeism, that can also mean major savings. But what about creativity? T'ai Chi's meditative quality enables practitioners to become more creative as they let go of being locked into old patterns. A popular corporate expression is to "think outside the box," which means to look beyond the established way of doing things, to try to find new and innovative approaches, capitalizing on constantly changing tools and technology. It's a useful concept, but how do we really think outside the box? We have to release the old ways of doing things. Again, T'ai Chi is about letting go of everything, mentally, emotionally, and physically which requires releasing prejudices and preconceptions, making us clearer and more open to new possibilities and potential. If T'ai Chi can help employees think outside the box, this will open them up to fresh innovative approaches and may boost profits more than anything we could begin to measure.

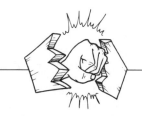

A T'ai Chi Punch Line

A community college near Kansas City provides T'ai Chi classes as a wellness program to their staff, and many participants are finding alleviation of chronic pain conditions, less stress, and fewer sick days. T'ai Chi is rapidly becoming the most popular wellness program for many companies. Isn't it great that companies are realizing that what is good for the employee is good for the company's profits as well?

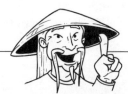

Sage Sifu Says

Albert Einstein said, "Imagination is more important than knowledge." When T'ai Chi and QiGong help us let go of physical, emotional, and mental tension, it literally expands our "imagination muscle." As we let go of old patterns, we open up to new and exciting concepts that our old, tense bodies and minds couldn't comprehend. We learn more easily and are more creative in using what we learn.

Lower Back Problems and Carpal Tunnel

Lower back problems are a large part of costly, unscheduled absenteeism. T'ai Chi is very effective at helping with chronic lower back pain, as well as other chronic pain problems.

Since T'ai Chi is the very best balance training in the world, causing participants to be half as likely to suffer falling injuries as others, T'ai Chi can reduce workplace injuries dramatically. Tell your company's Safety Director to look into the Emory University T'ai Chi study on balance. It will get his or her attention.

Some T'ai Chi exercises are very similar to exercises designed to prevent Repetitive Stress Injury, such as Carpal Tunnel Syndrome. Therefore, you may be hitting several birds with your well-thrown T'ai Chi stone.

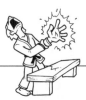

Ouch!

Even though QiGong can be done at your desk, it is also good to take breaks away from the workstation, in a quiet board room or the rest room, where you can do T'ai Chi in relative silence. Then when you return to your workstation, the QiGong will be even more effective, as if you brought some of the silence with you.

T'ai Chi's a Natural for the Office

One thing that makes T'ai Chi uniquely ideal for the workplace is that it requires no special clothing or equipment. If you have 15 minutes and a quiet room, you are all set to experience some amazing stress reduction and energy boosting.

Since T'ai Chi is so slow and gentle, you often need not work up a sweat when taking a T'ai Chi break. By simply loosening your tie or kicking off your heels, you are all set. In fact, Sitting QiGong or simple Moving QiGong can be done right at your desk. As employees become more adept at these tools of breath and relaxation, they'll use them throughout the day to reduce stress and boost performance.

Notice by simply kicking off your heels and loosening your tie, you are "suited" up for a T'ai Chi break.

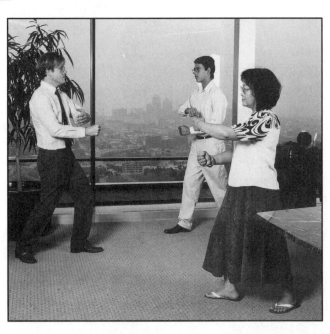

Internal Flexibility Makes Work Flexible

What your coworkers and you will soon discover is that the more loose and flexible you are physically, the more flexible you will become in your social and business interactions.

We literally hold onto prejudices, grudges, and resistance to change in our body's tight muscles. We cannot open our minds if we don't allow our bodies to loosen up. T'ai Chi's promotion of deep loosening and relaxed motion promotes a letting go of the control issues we all have. It can facilitate a looser, yet more productive work environment as communication becomes easier between employees who less and less resemble walking, emotional land mines.

T'ai Chi diffuses the stress bombs that build up within us and can make the workplace not only less dangerous, *but more fun.* We can discover the "real person" in our coworkers as their rigid armor begins to fall away. Part of that "realness" is the fun part of ourselves we were in touch with as kids. A rigid workplace environment can hide that fun, more vulnerable part of us. Therefore, T'ai Chi may not only help us enjoy our work more, but the company of our coworkers as well. Again, the Chinese say T'ai Chi helps return us to that magical youthful state of mind, which is not childish but *child-like.*

Office Politics and the "Great Corporate Cosmos"

Most companies are painfully aware that the machinations of office politics are a severe drain on productivity. On a personal level, most of us are all too familiar with the energy drain that office politics can cause.

The intra-office political maneuvering we often call office politics, which involves employees wasting time trying to alter office opinion of others through gossip or innuendo, is mostly rooted in fear and control issues. The more relaxed and at ease we are with ourselves, the more at ease we will be with coworkers, rather than reading our fear into office relationships. Again, T'ai Chi exercises not only help cleanse our mind and heart of rootless fears, but can help us let go of control issues. T'ai Chi's exercises, when done correctly, help us let go of attachment to outcome or destination, and just learn to flow through more effortless changes.

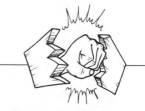

A T'ai Chi Punch Line

I worked as a human resources administrator for several years and came to realize that most employee problems are stress related. The more that HR departments can provide employees with stress management tools like T'ai Chi, the quieter things will be on the front lines of the HR office. Some employees have commented that when disagreements arise, whether they are between employees or between employees and management, T'ai Chi's calming influence made a constructive exchange of differing opinions possible.

T'ai Chi helps us to break from unhealthy patterns of internal fear or stress responses, and this can resonate out to the office relationships, helping us and our coworkers be both calmer and more productive. Just as tension begets tension, calm can help beget calm in those around us.

Imagine if employees used their one hour lunches not to gossip and politic themselves into a tension frenzy, but to do T'ai Chi for 25 minutes before lunch. Twenty-five minutes of breath and flowing relaxed motion could make the company and the world a vastly different place.

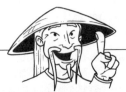

Sage Sifu Says

Rather than talking about work stuff at lunch, try taking a break from it all. If you have an hour lunch, do T'ai Chi for half an hour before lunch or, if you have only half an hour, take 15 minutes. This will help your mind and body disconnect from whatever problems you may face at work.

On the other hand, if you truly do not like your job, the quiet mindfulness that T'ai Chi offers can help you come to terms with it. Its focusing aspect may help you decide what you want, how to get it, and how to be calm and poised enough to perform a great interview for the job you do want. Then someone who really does want your job can come along and fill it, and the great flowing energy of the corporate cosmos can do its thing.

Ideas for Incorporating T'ai Chi into Your Workplace

T'ai Chi encourages us to let go of old ways and patterns while opening us to new, better ways of doing things. As discussed earlier, T'ai Chi can help us to think outside the box, to be open to fresh, innovative approaches. This is how T'ai Chi is being introduced to the workplace. Each company is doing it their own way and finding out how to use T'ai Chi's tools to fit their needs. Below are several sections on the nuts and bolts of making T'ai Chi part of your company's wellness program. If you are not the Wellness Director, bring this section to him or her.

Costs

Costs can vary widely. If you are a Wellness Director, the important thing to remember is that cheaper is not better. If you get a cut rate T'ai Chi program that few employees take advantage of, then you are not really saving your company any money. If absenteeism or disciplinary problems decline or productivity increases after the introduction of a T'ai Chi class at your company, then your company will profit in the long run. It is therefore in your best interest to find a good T'ai Chi instructor, one who is knowledgeable, approachable, and fun, and who can connect daily work stresses to his or her T'ai Chi instruction approach.

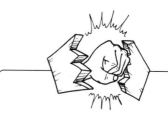

A T'ai Chi Punch Line

Many health insurance companies are now subsidizing or covering the cost of T'ai Chi and/or QiGong classes. Contact your carrier to find out if they do or ask them to if they do not.

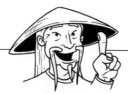

Sage Sifu Says

When possible, try taking a 15-minute T'ai Chi break before any major discussion or disagreement with a boss, employee, or coworker. Let go of all the reasons, justifications, or accusations associated with the issue as you let go of every muscle with each sighing exhale. In fact, let go of the issue entirely. When you come back to it, you will likely approach the problem in a much more comprehensively beneficial way that will more likely leave all parties winning.

Ways Companies Invest in T'ai Chi Programs

There are several ways companies can invest in T'ai Chi. Some companies passively promote T'ai Chi, offering a space for employees to practice during lunch or after work. Others do much more.

The best T'ai Chi and Stress Management seminars are optional. Provide employees with the option of working or attending the seminar, but do not make the seminar mandatory. Most people will opt for the seminar to get a break from work anyway, but the quality of the seminar is completely different if the employee has chosen to be there. This is the first step in an employee creating his or her own healthy lifestyle. If it's someone else's idea, we resist, but if we feel empowered to change ourselves, we have a vested interest in a positive outcome.

For example, company investment in a full stress management consulting program maximizes the benefits T'ai Chi offers. This usually involves a two-day program of about three hours per day, whereby the presenter gives an in-depth introduction to T'ai Chi and QiGong to prepare employees and the HR or Wellness Department to carry weekly classes.

This can lead to daily morning or afternoon T'ai Chi breaks, provided in a vacant boardroom, for example. Some companies may reward T'ai Chi practitioners with a 30-minute morning break, if instead of drinking coffee and sodas for 15 minutes, they use the 30-minute break to attend morning T'ai Chi classes in the area provided. This could be done in conjunction with a weekly one-hour video or live T'ai Chi class during lunch or after work.

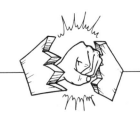

A T'ai Chi Punch Line

British dominance of the seas in the 1700s can, in part, be linked to the simple discovery that citrus fruits cure scurvy. Feeding British sailors limes, therefore, made it possible for British ships to stay at sea for much longer missions than enemy ships. Today's captains of industry who realize that stress is the greatest threat *to their crews* and who give their people tools like T'ai Chi to avoid illness and burnout will dominate in business.

For the daily T'ai Chi breaks, sign-in sheets could be used to document employee participation. This information may be helpful to acquire rebates or subsidies from company health insurance providers to cover the cost of T'ai Chi classes. Ask your carrier.

Also, it is good to collect testimonials from employees from time to time, as these usually list a myriad of health benefits each person gets from T'ai Chi, which also could be passed on to health insurance providers.

Other ways to offer company classes:

➤ Company investment in T'ai Chi classes by local instructors

➤ Company splits cost of classes in varying ratios with employees

➤ Company provides space and contacts instructor, but leaves payment up to employees

➤ Company cosponsors one-time introductory seminar with instructor and then allows instructor to recruit for community classes off-site from company

➤ On-site company classes are usually held before work, during lunch, or immediately after work. Companies are wise to consider offering employees who participate a half hour of paid time to participate in class.

For example, if employees attend a morning class, have half of the class start before work and half during paid work time. The potential savings in employee health, productivity, and attitude will more than make up for the minimal investment of the half hour of pay. Companies can thereby take the lead in encouraging employees to take up healthful habits that in turn promote decreased absenteeism, increased productivity, and diminished disciplinary problems.

The Least You Need to Know

➤ "Tie"-Chi can save companies big money.

➤ T'ai Chi can be done in work clothes in an office.

➤ T'ai Chi can help employees get along.

➤ Show this book to your Wellness Director, and you might get free classes at work.

➤ Companies can increase productivity by offering T'ai Chi classes to their employees.

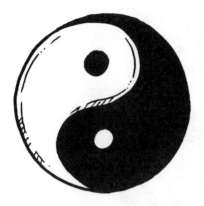

T'ai Chi's Philosophy of Balance and Flow

T'ai Chi is not an end in itself. T'ai Chi is a passageway to a healthier lifestyle. Dietary changes, the inclusion of regular massage therapy, acupuncture tune ups, and the power of positive thinking can all catapult you forward into even greater rewards that T'ai Chi offers. This chapter will expose you to many interesting and wonderful tools to further your life adventure in self-awareness and limitless growth.

The Yin Yang of Diet

T'ai Chi's movements are a blend of hard and soft, exertion and relaxation, force and yielding. In fact, the T'ai Chi symbol is the yin/yang symbol—the symbol of balance. Just as T'ai Chi and QiGong are built upon the concepts of balance, so is every other aspect of healthy living. Chinese cooking adheres to these same principles.

In Chinese cooking, a good cook balances the use of yin foods and yang foods to create a meal that is not only delicious, but provides optimum health benefits. In a way, a good Chinese chef is almost like a pharmacist, blending nutrients, herbs, and Qi into a prescription that treats the eyes, palate, and health.

This ancient yin/yang symbol is actually called "T'ai Chi." It represents two things: that everything in the universe exists within each individual thing (even you), and that we should seek balance in all things.

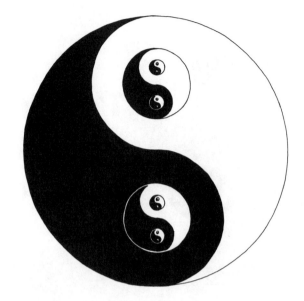

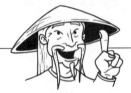

Sage Sifu Says

Many nutritionists see the Chinese diet as optimum, approximately 50 percent grain (rice), 30 percent vegetables, and 20 percent meat. Each person is unique, and our needs vary depending on our current health and activities. Ask your physician or a qualified dietician to discover your optimum diet.

Be aware that just eating Chinese food does not mean a healthy diet. There are healthy and unhealthy Chinese foods as well. Stick to stir fried rather than batter fried meat and vegetables. Steamed fish is excellent. Use your own good judgement.

Green vegetables are yin food. They are cool and easily digested and are helpful for certain parts and functions of the body. Meat is a yang food. Yang is power and provides great energy to the body, but is less easily digested. Chinese herbs are divided into cool and hot, dry and wet, each of which is good for certain conditions. There are many good books on Chinese herbs. Again, your food becomes not only a culinary treat but also a prescription for optimum health.

Chinese Herbs & Teas for Conditions

Ginseng tea is made from ginseng root. The roots resemble a person's head and body. Ginseng has yang qualities. If a person's condition is overly yin, or cool and damp, an herbalist may suggest herbs promoting the yang qualities of dry and hot. For example, fresh ginger tea may be good to treat some early cold symptoms. Bitter melon soup, a yin food, may be used to treat an overactive yang condition like nosebleeds. Consult a qualified herbalist for more detailed information. Make sure your physician is aware of any herbal therapy you may engage in.

Feng Shui: Architectural T'ai Chi

The Chinese believe that Qi, or life energy, not only flows through living things but through all things. According to this belief, we move in a great ocean of invisible energy that affects and interacts with energy from other beings, nature, and even buildings. In fact, they have developed an architectural system to affect the way energy flows through your home or business in order to maximize health, happiness, and prosperity. Feng Shui is like architectural T'ai Chi, or T'ai Chi for your house.

Have you ever noticed how almost all Chinese restaurants have aquariums and many near the front door? This arrangement is based on Feng Shui. Running water is very good for the room's Qi.

Western architecture often uses running water for decorative purposes, but science is now suggesting that the use of water in architecture is also functional. Many homes and geographical areas are bombarded by positive ions in the air. This can aggravate allergies or cause other physiological or mental discomforts. Some of this positive ion overload is because of modern electricity, but some is a

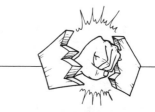

A T'ai Chi Punch Line

My wife was two weeks overdue with our first son when we went to eat at a family-owned Chinese restaurant where we were friends with the owners. When the owner discovered that my wife was overdue, she said, "Wait here, I get something just for you." She came back with a special "black sesame" drink for my wife. The owner said, "Tonight you will have the baby." We laughed, but about six hours later, my wife went into labor.

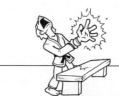

Ouch!

The Chinese health philosophy frowns on iced drinks because they introduce too much yin into the body too quickly. This shocks the body and upsets the balance. Hot or tepid drinks are preferred because the body is naturally warm.

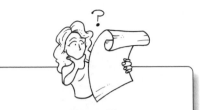

Know Your Chinese

Feng Shui means "wind" and "water." Wind represents universal forces, while water represents earth forces. Balancing the two creates optimum health and prosperity.

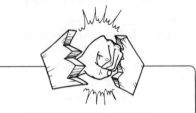

A T'ai Chi Punch Line

Donald Trump incorporates Feng Shui into the architectural design of all of the buildings he constructs or remodels.

natural phenomenon. Running water produces negative ions, which can balance the ions in a room, home, or business, making it more pleasant and more healthful. If a restaurant makes you feel more at ease, you will likely come back there more often, making the restaurant more prosperous. So, Feng Shui works on principles based on a subatomic understanding of the energy dynamics in a room, which in the end can lead to a happier, more prosperous existence.

The I-Ching

As you learned in Part 4 on the Kuang Ping Yang style of T'ai Chi, which has 64 forms, there are 64 possible combinations of hexagrams in the I-Ching.

There are many ways to use the I-Ching, and there is some debate about how or what it really does. Some think it is a fortune-telling device, while others see it as a tool for self-analysis or contemplation of self. There are 64 possible hexagrams, which represent all the possible ways life can transform.

Some modern analysts compare the hexagram system of the I-Ching to the Rorschach Test, where the person reading the hexagrams is really defined by how he or she sees them. To read your I-Ching, you throw the hexagrams out, or shake yarrow sticks from a cup, and the way they fall tells you what to look up. There are books that list the hexagrams meanings. They are often just vague enough so that you must interpret for yourself the detailed meaning for your life. Therefore, when we use this method of divination we are compelled to introspection, to understand who we are, what we want, and where we want to go in life. Seen in this light, the I-Ching can be a very healthful and potentially invaluable tool. Some bookstores will have books, or even kits, so that you can practice using the I-Ching system yourself.

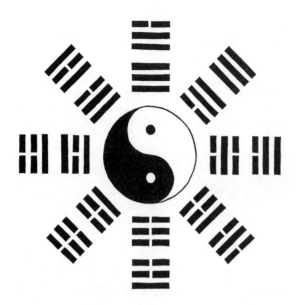

The 64 possible hexagram combinations represent all the possible forms of life's changes, just as styles of T'ai Chi with 64 movements represent possible physical changes we go through.

Rest and Rejuvenation

The yin and yang symbol of T'ai Chi symbolizes that we must balance our natures in our bodies and in the world around us. In our modern fast-paced lives, we are too reliant on busyness and constant noise. We consider television to be a form of relaxation. Actually a small amount can be, but the hours of television watching most Americans do is actually unhealthy. In fact, the American Medical Association has stated that over two hours per day is unhealthy.

Just as activity is important to our health, so is absolute rest. Most of us probably find it difficult just to sit, to simply be and serenely enjoy the absence of stimulation. At first, the slowness and quiet quality of T'ai Chi and QiGong drive many people a little nuts.

This is a cleansing process. The more anxiety we feel, breathe through, and let go of, the more we settle into a clarity and calmness that we eventually learn to enjoy. By sitting still we become aware of anxieties and tensions that we may have buried in our subconscious mind. These repressed feelings can manifest as muscle tension, asthma attacks, volatile emotions, and so on, unless we become aware of them, feel them, and then begin to breathe through them by physically letting the

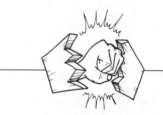

A T'ai Chi Punch Line

One day my wife and I went to a temple in Hong Kong, and while there had our fortunes forecast by a priest using the I-Ching. After divining our fortune, the priest told my wife, "You are pregnant." We laughed because we knew that we had been careful. Two days later, my wife got dizzy, so we rushed her to a clinic where the doctor did blood tests. The doctor came back and announced, "You are pregnant."

muscles let go and the mind relax. The cleansing pleasure of that "empty awareness" is perhaps the most healthful thing we can do for ourselves. It gives our mind a chance to rest, to heal, and to recharge. This also gives our spiritual nature an opportunity to come forth. We can get a new perspective on life, just by sitting. Just as a drug addict must go through a period of anxiety to let go of the craving for drugs, those of us that are addicted to "busyness" and constant stimulation (TV or whatever) must go through that anxiety period. But eventually we touch into the bliss of stillness of mind.

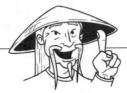

Sage Sifu Says

A famous Vietnamese monk once said that we are like glasses of dirty water. Each day the dirt gets shook up, and we become cloudy and unclear. If we take time to sit still, our stress settles down, and we again can see clearly.

T'ai Chi Teaches Mindful Living

T'ai Chi's slow process and seemingly endless progression from one movement to the next teaches us to let go of outcome and be in the moment. In the West, we call this "stopping to smell the roses." With T'ai Chi, we don't just think about stopping to smell the roses. We simply must do it. You cannot stand to perform a 20-minute slow-motion exercise like T'ai Chi and stay in a rush-rush-hurry-hurry mentality. It is impossible. Therefore T'ai Chi is like a magic formula that actually changes who you are. Its methodology forces us to love the act of living, just as we must love the feel, the sensation, the breath, and the motion of each T'ai Chi movement, so that we don't anxiously wait for it to be over. Life becomes a sacrament, every moment, and every person we touch becomes sacred and a miracle. As T'ai Chi's slow mindfulness causes us to subtly attune to the miracle of our own existence, we see the world around as miraculous. On a physical level as we daily immerse ourselves in Qi, or life's energy, we connect with that quality in all living things.

The mindful living that T'ai Chi teaches spills out into every aspect of our lives. The following is a list of exercises you can perform to bring T'ai Chi's mindfulness into every aspect of your life.

➤ When you take a sip of lime-water or hot tea, really smell the rich odor as you drink. Let the aroma fill your awareness.

➤ Feel that sip as it's in your mouth. As you swallow it, feel the heat or cold go down your throat. Experience its descent all the way into your stomach.

➤ When you hold a hot cup of tea, watch the steam rise. Get your face right up next to it. The steam is agitated atoms that burst free of the surface and scream outward into space, just like the huge bursts that erupt from the surface of the sun. Enjoy this fabulous display of erupting atoms.

➤ Simplify your diet, drinking more water with a lime twist and less soda or beer. Take the time to really taste and smell the lime. Lime is an exquisite gift we've been given. Usually we must drink very sweet over-flavored things because we don't slow down enough to really taste them. So we need the shock value of 13 sugar cubes and the other sticky stuff that come in most cans of soda.

➤ Eat more fruit and vegetables. Really stop and chew them. Feel their texture, their temperature, and savor their subtle flavor and smell.

➤ When you cook, feel the food as you cut it up. Listen to the sizzling as it cooks and really smell the richness of its aroma. Pretend for a moment that this was your last day on earth, and you would never be able to smell these smells, hear these sounds, or taste these tastes again.

➤ Sit and watch nature. Nature cannot be analyzed or fixed. Nature simply washes over you. Watch the clouds move, the trees sway, and the weather unfold. This world is a miracle placed here for your enjoyment. Don't take its beauty for granted.

➤ When your spouse or children talk to you, just listen. Observe their faces, the excitement in their voices. Let the images of their day wash over your mind. Do not worry about how you are "supposed" to respond. Enjoy their presence.

➤ Observe people, experience them. Imagine for a moment that you were the only person on earth, and there was never ever going to be anyone else but you. You probably would be filled with desire to speak to others, to enjoy their existence. Here they are, enjoy.

➤ Let life wash over you. Do what needs to be done, whether its washing dishes or paying bills with a sense of unhurried pleasure, like T'ai Chi movements are done. If we don't run from what we must do, it can be pleasant, and all things simply work out, as if we did nothing at all.

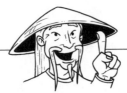

Sage Sifu Says

The T'ai Chi symbol, or yin/yang symbol, literally means the supreme ultimate point in the universe. When you follow the suggestions to allow T'ai Chi to weave it's mindfulness into your life, you begin to feel more and more as though you are in the center of the universe.

The Least You Need to Know

➤ Balance your diet, like your life.

➤ "Fresh" ginger tea at the first sign of a cold.

➤ Open, flowing interior design does much more than just look good.

➤ I-Ching games can help you understand yourself better.

➤ T'ai Chi teaches savoring life and smelling the roses.

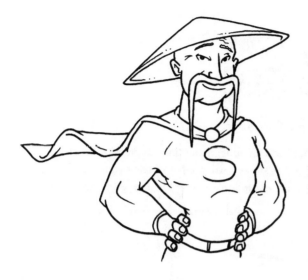

Chapter 27

Do T'ai Chi: Change the World

In this Chapter

➤ How T'ai Chi can lower unemployment

➤ T'ai Chi lowers health care costs

➤ How T'ai Chi is helping schools

➤ T'ai Chi may reduce crime and violence

➤ T'ai Chi can help clean up the environment and heal our world

---

T'ai Chi is widely misunderstood. Is it an exercise, a martial art, or a meditation *technique*? Actually, T'ai Chi is all those things, but it also offers so much more. T'ai Chi can be a key to discovering our personal empowerment. As we find that we can take control over our body's circulation, our blood pressure, and our stress responses, we are empowered. This empowerment begins to resonate out to every aspect of our lives, work, relationships, and society.

As we feel empowered and T'ai Chi works its clarifying magic, we find learning easier and more exciting. We become drawn to learning as the world becomes fresher and more magical due to our new attitude of well-being. T'ai Chi cultivates and supports our childlikeness, our curiosity, and our zest for life.

T'ai Chi also teaches us how precious and miraculous life can be. When we treasure each moment of our lives, we are much less likely to engage in acts that endanger our health or our freedom. When we feel at peace within ourselves, we are much less likely to hurt others. Much violence is the act of someone in personal pain who externalizes that pain on others. T'ai Chi can help heal that pain, thereby reducing much violence.

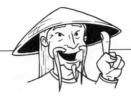

Sage Sifu Says

To get the maximum benefits from T'ai Chi and QiGong, make time to practice them every day. After a while it won't be a chore at all. You will relish and savor your T'ai Chi moments, looking forward to them like a school kid looks forward to the weekend.

T'ai Chi and Unemployment

Since people who grew up in high-stress households have higher unemployment rates, T'ai Chi may help both parents and children change that pattern. Secondly, since many people are increasingly required by the modern economy to change careers several times, T'ai Chi's promotion of letting go of the past and relaxing into change can be helpful to adults in today's job market.

Children's Stress Can Reduce Their Employability

England's Royal Academy of Pediatrics College released a study that concluded that "stressful" households caused problems for children that could last a lifetime. One thing they discovered was that children from such households endured higher unemployment levels than kids from more peaceful households. We know that stress limits our creativity and can affect our self-esteem. T'ai Chi's ability to provide children with a tool that can help them find a calm place within, even when home is "less than calm," can be of powerful help to them.

T'ai Chi Is Relaxing into the Future

In today's modern workforce, it is estimated that most of us will change, not jobs, but careers over five times in our lifetime. For people who find change difficult, this can be excruciatingly stressful and even life threatening over time. In a world of constant and relentless change, T'ai Chi's ability to help us mentally, emotionally, and physically let go can be a great help.

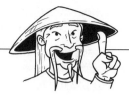

Sage Sifu Says

Change in and of itself is an essential and wonderful part of life. Our unhealthy responses to change are the problem. Again, T'ai Chi is a tool to lubricate our way into the challenging and exciting future that awaits those who rise to the occasion.

By being able to let go of past employment and being open to new information and self-definitions, we can be ready to flow into our next occupation. This flowing can happen, not only less stressfully, but with an adventurous anticipation, just like when we were kids. This is what T'ai Chi can help us do as individuals and as a society.

When you catch yourself considering worst-case scenarios while engaged in a task or project, take a deep breath and let your entire body release thoughts, tensions, and fears. Then make a list or flow chart of what is required for success. This will let you realistically decide whether to proceed rather than resist change because of irrational fears. T'ai Chi promotes a sense of being in the moment, of dealing with the tasks at hand, and of letting go of fear-based projections of the future.

T'ai Chi and the Health Care Crisis

Approximately 80 percent of the illnesses that send us to the doctor are due to stress. The six leading causes of death are stress related. Our health care crisis is literally due to stress. Stress can be managed, and there is perhaps no more effective stress management tool than daily T'ai Chi and QiGong meditations.

Hospitals and insurance carriers are beginning to incorporate T'ai Chi and QiGong into what they offer clients. Physicians from neurologists, to cardiac and hypertension specialists, to mental health providers are prescribing T'ai Chi for a host of physical, emotional, and mental conditions. Medical university nursing programs are also introducing T'ai Chi to their students as part of their training. Others schools are considering offering it to all medical students.

T'ai Chi begins to show us that we have a health care crisis simply because we choose to have a health care crisis. Each of us has it within our own power to dramatically lower our dependence on general health care, pharmacology, and surgery. The fastest growing investment industry in the U.S. today is pharmaceuticals. The top three are ulcer, high blood pressure, and mood altering medications. T'ai Chi and/or QiGong can have significantly positive effects on all three of these conditions in some cases.

T'ai Chi and QiGong are not at odds with modern Western health care. They can be partners with it. You don't decide between medication or surgery, and T'ai Chi. If you need medication or surgery, then use it. However, medication and surgery should not be our first line of defense. If we practice T'ai Chi, we may never develop the need for certain medications or for much heart surgery. Again, stress is the reason most of the physical conditions requiring medication or surgery develop in the first place. If we daily water our "T'ai Tree" roots with the soothing balm of life energy, we will be less likely to ever need that medication or surgery, saving ourselves pain and money, while saving our society a great financial burden. We cannot afford to ignore our body's signals and our health until we are in a crisis situation and then expect society to lavish money upon us for expensive surgery or medication. This isn't just about Medicare alone; *all* our health insurance premiums are sky rocketing due to a national need to become mindful of our health. T'ai Chi can save us all big money and help us feel good while doing it.

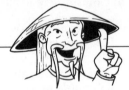

Sage Sifu Says

When going to the doctor, think less of expecting the doctor to "heal you." Rather, think in terms of you and the doctor in partnership. Ask the doctor what healthful habits or activities you can engage in to facilitate your healing. The question should be, "How can I heal me?"

T'ai Chi in Education

Studies show that change, even change for the better, is stressful. A good example is when you upgrade your computer. The newer program gives you new tools to make your work faster and more efficient, but letting go of the old ways and learning the new is often stressful.

So, each day our children in many ways are learning new ways to do everything, both at home and at school. Kid's today are under tremendous stress because the world is changing very fast, and they will see changes we never dreamed of in our lives. Therefore, the best tool they can be given to launch out upon the world with confidence and health is, you guessed it, T'ai Chi.

T'ai Chi Helps Students Stay Current, Even in a Fast Current

Remember how T'ai Chi brings you back to the calm center no matter how fast life's carousel is spinning. In today's rapidly changing world, this is a very important tool to give our children. No matter how much math, science, and economic facts we give them, they will be lost if they don't know how to thrive healthfully in a world of change. Why? Because our understanding of math, science and economics is changing on an almost daily basis. Of all the discoveries made since the inception of man, nearly all have been made in our lifetimes, and the world is only getting faster with the explosion of the information age. Therefore, a child with mind/body training that can help them adapt to new ways easier and more healthfully, will have a distinct advantage over kids *who only learn* the current ways things are done, or the current text books facts.

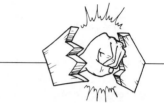

A T'ai Chi Punch Line

If you look at many long-term T'ai Chi practitioners, Chinese or Western, you will find very vibrant people, often at the pinnacles of their professions. T'ai Chi practitioners do not fear and run from change, but find it essential to a full life.

If you refer back to the "Stress Is the Symptom" section in Chapter 3, you'll see that we too often respond to stressors (like change) in an unhealthy way. When this happens chronically, it can even inhibit our thinking processes, literally shrinking parts of the brain. So, by teaching T'ai Chi, we help children calm, provide them a physical model to relax through changes, which thereby can improve their mental function.

T'ai Chi Is Health Study from the Inside Out

Hopefully every school will eventually provide T'ai Chi instruction through all levels of education and to teachers as well. Teaching universities are beginning to incorporate it into their advanced credit offerings for teachers at all levels, and many teachers are finding T'ai Chi on their own to deal with personal stress from overcrowded classrooms and low education budgets. T'ai Chi is a cross between physical education and health science. It may eventually become a staple of health science. What better way for kids to learn about their body and health than by paying attention to the laboratory they walk around in every day, their own miraculous minds and bodies, through practicing T'ai Chi's mindful exercises.

Although most of the high school T'ai Chi classes I've taught have been in health science, physical education, art, and drama, instructors are considering T'ai Chi as an adjunct to their classes.

T'ai Chi Can Help Students Avoid Drugs

Some schools are already providing T'ai Chi to students. I have personally taught T'ai Chi and QiGong relaxation therapy to students in the elementary, junior high, high school, and university level through health science, college preparatory programs, and drug abuse prevention programs. Health science teachers have told me that students claim the main reason they begin smoking or using drugs and alcohol is to alleviate stress. Of course, those of us with more life experience know that in the end, drug abuse creates more stress, but it is not enough to simply tell kids to "just say no." We must take the next step and provide them with tools to manage the enormous stress they face in an increasingly complex world.

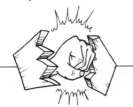

A T'ai Chi Punch Line

Many people using T'ai Chi to rehabilitate from drug abuse problems like the fact that T'ai Chi gives them something to replace the old habits with. Rather than just denying themselves the high they loved, they are growing toward a new life as T'ai Chi helps them improve each and every day.

T'ai Chi and Crime

T'ai Chi is now being taught in prison, as well as in court-sponsored rehabilitation programs. T'ai Chi's ability to build self-esteem, heal childhood trauma, and manage potentially violent stress makes it an incredible coping tool for anyone trying to change. If we want to reduce crime, finding ways people can become productive parts of society is a cost-effective and just plain effective way to do it. It costs twice as much to send a child to prison as it does to send that child to Harvard. The United States has incarcerated more of its children than any nation in the world, per capita. It is time to find creative solutions like T'ai Chi and mind/body fitness training to heal the very roots of crime—*the potential criminals*. To do this before the crime occurs will save us all much pain and vast amounts of money.

T'ai Chi and Law Enforcement

Law enforcement officers work in constant danger and often see only the worst sides of people. This can be very stressful. Historically, stress-related maladies like alcoholism, drug abuse, coronary heart disease, diabetes, and suicide have been problems within law enforcement, according to *Police Chief Magazine* and the US Public Health Service. T'ai Chi may be an effective multipurpose way to help law enforcement officers deal with job-related stress. T'ai Chi's martial applications would be an added bonus to officers learning T'ai Chi's soothing stress-management tools. T'ai Chi can help in several ways. First, it can help officers dump job stress after work. Then if they do go out for a drink after T'ai Chi class, they will be doing it for pleasure, rather than for stress reduction. This can mean the difference between a couple of social drinks and a mind-numbing binge.

Second, if officers are less stressed on duty, they will likely see more options in any given situation. Problems can be diffused more easily when in a calmer, clearer state. Even in difficult situations, T'ai Chi's calming effects can resonate, especially if it helps the officers sleep better, which T'ai Chi is known to do. So T'ai Chi's calming aspects can help diffuse potentially dangerous situations, which leaves the officer with less stress to take off duty. Less stress begets less stress, and so on and so on.

T'ai Sci

Some therapists are beginning to direct their patients to T'ai Chi classes to learn how to diffuse their stress in a more healthful way.

Hopefully, departments will eventually provide officers with seven-hour shifts and use the last hour for T'ai Chi decompression time. This will make business sense for all the reasons listed in the chapter on corporate T'ai Chi, but these benefits are magnified since law enforcement's stress can be even higher.

T'ai Chi and Violence

This sounds strange, but most domestic violence is a very ineffective form of stress management. Domestic violence is a way that a very unhappy person takes out their personal stress on their loved ones. It's ineffective because as we tear down those around us, that eventually tears us down. We create a sanctuary of pain rather than a loving home.

T'ai Chi can change that from many angles. If children begin to use T'ai Chi's mind/body fitness stress-management tools to self-heal in school, the cycle of pain at home will be changed and diminished in some ways. Then if parents can be encouraged to learn these tools through community services, they will change the cycle even more effectively. There is a great spider web of connection in a community that will be affected as well. If one parent breaks a cycle of abuse and pain, his or her children will not spread that pain by being mean to the children around them at school. Or by growing up and passing it down to their kids by being violent to them.

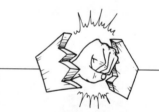

A T'ai Chi Punch Line

Many T'ai Chi practitioners hear others tell them they have "changed," "are calmer," or "are easier to be around," before they even notice the changes in themselves. Even when you are feeling stress, others may see you as "mellow" in comparison to the rest of the world.

Alcohol or other substance abuse aggravate much domestic violence. The benefits of T'ai Chi for drug rehabilitation is discussed in Chapter 24.

There is a famous "kick the cat" story which shows how a community is affected by one person's calm or rage.

An executive gets a traffic ticket on the way to work and then fumes at his administrative assistant. She in turn snaps at the other executives and employees she deals with. They get ticked off and snap at their coworkers, who are testy with people in the other companies they deal with on the phone, and so on. Eventually thousands of people who have had a lousy day hit the freeway and begin to give the one-fingered salute to other motorists. And so it goes.

Finally all these seething people get home and yell at their spouses, who yell at the kids, who walk upstairs and kick the cat.

T'ai Chi can inverse this process ending up with thousands of family cats getting a loving caress by kids growing up in a more loving world, nurtured by parents who work at companies that provide health tools to them like T'ai Chi. Sound far-fetched? Not really. Stress is the source of much of our communal pain, and stress management like T'ai Chi is a balm that can dramatically heal it.

A study done by the Transcendental Meditation Foundation (which teaches an excellent form of stress management called TM) found that when a small percentage of the population of a community, school, or organization practiced TM, it had a positive impact on that entire social body.

Therefore, even though most people will never practice T'ai Chi, the few that do may change the entire community in positive ways.

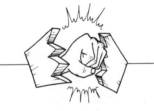

A T'ai Chi Punch Line

Once you learn T'ai Chi, you'll begin to notice people practicing everywhere you go, in any country in the world. T'ai Chi is an international language. My students have done T'ai Chi with people in England, France, Japan, Vietnam, Mexico, China, El Salvador, and Cuba, to name a few. As you travel, T'ai Chi will give you a pleasant vehicle to interact with and meet other people, even if you don't speak their language.

T'ai Chi and the Environment

At first, it may not seem like T'ai Chi has anything to do with our world's environment, but it does. The word *T'ai Chi* means the Supreme Ultimate Point in the Universe. This means that every single part of the entire world exists within each and every thing, even you and me. Modern physics demonstrates this by explaining that all things are made of energy, *the same energy*. You, I, the sun and moon, and earth's oceans and mountains are all made of the same energy. We are connected. This is brought home even more as science explains that you and I and everyone on this planet has breathed an oxygen atom breathed by Jesus, Buddha, and Mohammed. The world gets smaller.

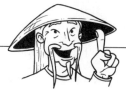

Sage Sifu Says

Each time you walk outside look up at the sky and at the trees or grass. Let the full breadth of nature's beauty wash over you. Think of opening your body to the universal energy as if you were an open airy sponge that could fill with the life around you, and likewise you can expand out to merge with it. If you make this a habit and take 30 or 60 seconds to do this each time you walk in or out of your home, it will change your life.

When you practice T'ai Chi and especially sitting QiGong, you often feel at peace, somehow connected to the world around you, as if you were the center of the universe. This experience leaves you feeling as though you matter, yet it also leaves us feeling as though every other person and every other thing in this world is of vast and profound importance as well.

T'ai Chi and QiGong reminds us that we are energy by immersing our mind and body in the experience of it each day. This constant immersion reminds us how closely we are linked to all things. This isn't an illusion. The illusion is that we think we are separate from the world. The rainforest and ocean are the earth's lungs and thermostats. Without them we perish. So, to feel "connected" to the world is to become real. T'ai Chi and QiGong help us to become more and more real.

Our decisions about how to live in our world will be healthfully influenced by the "realness" T'ai Chi cultivates. This will be a powerful asset to building a cleaner, healthier world. As mentioned in Part 1 of this book, T'ai Chi promotes a feeling of optimum mental, emotional, and physical health therapists call *homeostasis*. By tuning into that healthful center everyday, we are more drawn to ingesting healthful foods, water, and air, and therefore more conscious of the state of our small planet because this is where our water, food, and air come from.

As with all things, the world's environmental health begins with our own state of health. Your heart beats to supply oxygen to the entire body. However, the first thing the heart feeds is itself because if it is healthier, stronger, and clearer, it is more useful to it's world (our body). Therefore, by feeding yourself the healing force of life energy everyday, you enable yourself to be a healing force as you flow through the world *around you*.

> ### The Least You Need to Know
>
> ➤ T'ai Chi helps heal our society, our world, and us.
>
> ➤ T'ai Chi saves money in healthcare and may lower crime and unemployment rates.
>
> ➤ T'ai Chi helps us all "just get along."

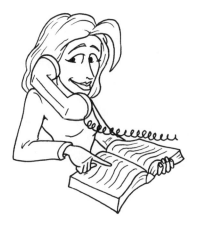

T'ai Chi Organizations and Energy Work Centers

There are many fine T'ai Chi and QiGong schools throughout the United States. Below is a short list of a few fine instructors or schools that the author has either personally worked with or been recommended to, followed by Web sources to assist you in locating more T'ai Chi and QiGong contacts and sources.

For those interested in an in-depth study of the life transforming tools of energy work, a listing of Actualism Centers can be found in the T'ai Chi instruction section. These are also highly recommended by the author, who began 20 years ago, and continues to study through the Coast Star Center of Actualism in Costa Mesa, California. Integrative, or natural medicine, is a great adjunct to your overall T'ai Chi lifestyle. Therefore, a short list of holistic health professionals from various fields are listed below. Again, the Web may be a good research resource for other integrative health professionals.

T'ai Chi

National Guang Ping Yang T'ai Chi Association
P.O. Box 1721, Nevada City, CA 95959
(415) 989-5665 (Northern California)
President, Henry Look

Pacific School of T'ai Chi and QiGong
Contact: Chris Luth (800) 266-5803

Peihong Luan
E-mail: mulantaiji@aol.com
Mulan Quan T'ai Chi Instruction (Los Angeles area)

The Qigong Research and Practice Center
P.O. Box 1727
Nederland, CO 80466
(303) 258-0971

Ken Cohen, an internationally renowned QiGong and T'ai Chi Ch'uan Master, whose work has been published in both China and the West, offers lectures, seminars, classes and educational materials.

Red Road Martial Arts
Contact: Sam Barnes (949) 640-7099
Email: Eeskah@aol.com
T'ai Chi, Taikuk Kwan, QiGong, and Push Hands (Orange County, CA)

Stress Management and Relaxation Technology (SMART)
P.O. Box 7786
Shawnee Mission, KS 66207-0786
(913) 648-2256 or (913) 648-CALM
www.taichismart.com

T'ai Chi and QiGong [energy work] Instruction: Kuang Ping Yang Style, Mulan Quan Basic, Mulan Quan Fan Style, & Mulan Quan Sword Style. Also, Corporate Consulting on Stress Management in the Workplace.

T'ai Chi Instruction
Contact: Colin Berg (425) 861-8658
E-mail: colinberg@earthlink.net
Kuang Ping Yang Style (Seattle)

Warrior of Light T'ai Chi Studio
(714) 536-9451 (Southern California)
Director: Jennifer Booth
Kuang Ping Yang Style and Sword Style

Web Sources

The Chinese Boxing Institute International
www.threedragons.com

Qi—The Journal of Traditional Chinese Health & Fitness
www.qi-journal.com

Traditional Chinese Medicine. Calendar of events for Traditional Chinese Medical Workshops and T'ai Chi events. Partial listings of T'ai Chi instructors nationwide and international.

For **Yang Style T'ai Chi in Canada**, contact:
www.chebucto.ns.ca/Philosophy/Taichi/contacts.html

You may find local classes in your area by going to America Online's Web search, AOL Netfind, and entering the keyword "tai chi" and then your city. There are national T'ai Chi organizations for most major styles, many of which may be located through the Internet.

Energy Work

Actualism centers offer in-depth training in energy work, which is rooted in the same ancient truths as QiGong and yogic energy healing. However, actualism is designed for the Western student and can make these sometimes esoteric concepts much more tangible and more useful to the Western student.

For more in-depth training in energy work, contact the following Actualism centers:

Coast Star Center
Costa Mesa, CA
(714) 957-9346
Co-Directors: Jennifer Booth/Alyssa Janus

Coast Star Center offers all Actualism services. From beginning through advanced energy work instruction to Body Work and training in performing Body Work. This center also offers acupuncture and T'ai Chi classes are held at a nearby studio.

Body Work is a massage therapy technique that involves external energy work methods whereby the client and therapist use their life energy tools to maximize the clearing and energizing potential of the physical tissue massage. You must have introductory energy work classes prior to receiving Body Work at actualism centers. All centers that offer Body Work also provide the introductory classes.

Escondido, CA Star Center
Escondido, CA
(619) 743-5240
Director: Alice Y. Stearns

Los Angeles Star Center
Los Angeles, CA
(213) 660-5283
Director: Stan Smith

This center offers beginning through advanced energy work instruction and Body Work.

New York Star Center
New York, NY
(212) 873-5826
Co-Directors: Dr. Bruce Jaffe/Bernice B. Cousins

New York classes are available from beginning to advanced levels.

San Diego Star Center
San Diego, CA
(619) 462-6570
Director: Penny Snyder

The San Diego center offers beginning through advanced energy work classes, Body Work sessions, and acupuncture.

Other Actualism Classes
For Actualism classes in San Francisco, Arizona, Montana, and other areas, call (800) 347-2460. Actualism's Web Page can be found at www.actualism.org/noframes-act.html.

Natural Health Centers

Acupuncture Society of America
(913) 931-0287
E-mail: ryenniedc@email.msn.com

The Acupuncture Society of America specializes in Traditional Chinese Medicine, offering acupuncture treatments and training throughout the U.S. Herbology, T'ui Na, T'ai Chi, and QiGong are also offered through their facility.

Integrative Medicine Clinic
2235 Thousand Oaks Drive, Suite 102
San Antonio, TX 78232
(210) 697-8585

The Integrative Medicine Clinic blends conventional and natural therapies for health and well-being.

Intergrative Acupuncture/Energy Work Practice
Contact: Linda Langhorn (760) 634-3803 (San Diego)

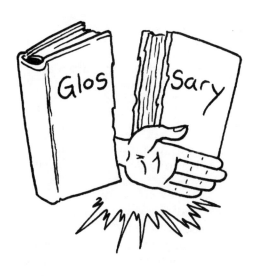

Glossary

Abdominal breathing   The QiGong breathing technique, whereby the abdominal area, or lower lungs fills first, then the upper chest, fully inflating the lungs. On the exhale, the upper chest relaxes inward as the lungs deflate, followed by the abdominal muscles relaxing inward allowing the lower lungs to deflate, fully expending the air from the lungs.

Acupressure   A massage technique of stimulating the acupuncture points without the use of acupuncture needles.

Acupuncture   A medical science that manipulates the flow of Qi, or life energy, through the body to maximize the body's health systems.

Acupuncture maps   Diagrams or models to help acupuncturists locate the acupuncture points on the body.

Aura   The sometimes visible aspect of life energy, whether through Kirlian photography or with the naked eye.

Biofeedback   A computer program often used to train people to relax under stress, by showing their blood pressure, heart rate, and so on, while the participant uses relaxation techniques to normalize those indicators.

Bone marrow cleansing   Moving QiGong exercise designed to cleanse the bone marrow of stress that might inhibit the immune system.

Carry the Moon   Moving QiGong exercise designed to help the spine stay supple, support kidney function, and promote flexibility throughout the frame.

Center   The physical, mental, emotional, and spiritual clarity that T'ai Chi and QiGong are designed to cultivate. Modern psychologists call this "homeostasis."

Chen style   An ancient T'ai Chi style and the basis of the Yang style.

The Chinese drum   A QiGong warm up for T'ai Chi preparation.

Chinese Medica   The bible of Traditional Chinese Medicine, encompassing all known knowledge on acupuncture, herbal medicine, and QiGong.

Crisis   The Chinese character for "crisis" is made of two characters, the character for "danger" plus the one for "opportunity."

Dan tien   The physical center of your body. An energy center approximately 1 $^1/_2$ to 3 inches below the navel near the center of the body.

DHEA   Adequate dehydroepiandrosterone levels are related to youthfulness and a more functional immune system. QiGong practice is believed to elevate DHEA levels.

Dong Gong   Moving QiGong.

Energy meridians   In Chinese "jing luo" or channel network. Modern acupuncturists may refer to them as "bioenergetic circuits." These are the paths that Qi moves through to circulate within the body, although they are not physical vessels like veins or arteries. They are energy channels where energy appears to flow more easily through the body's tissue. There are 14 main meridians, and 12 of those are directly associated with bodily organs; for example, heart, liver, and so on.

External QiGong   A Traditional Chinese Medical practice, whereby the provider allows his/her Qi, cultivated through internal QiGong practice, to flow, usually from their hands, out into the patient to help their healing process.

Fan lao huan tong   In Chinese this means "reverse old age and return to youthfulness"; the goal of T'ai Chi and QiGong.

Feng shui   The Chinese design art for creating flow and balance of energy within homes and other structures.

Fight or flight response   The body's reflex response to stress that involves elevated blood pressure, heart rate, and feelings of subdued panic.

Free radicals   Atoms with an extra electron, believed to contribute to the aging process. Regular T'ai Chi practice may reduce the cell damage these cause.

Grand Terminus   The yin-yang symbol, and also the final movement of the Kuang Ping Yang style of T'ai Chi.

Holistic   Chinese philosophy that sees the entire universe within each individual part, in much the same way that our body's building blocks of DNA coding is contained within each individual cell of our bodies.

Homeostasis   Modern therapists use this term to describe a chemical, emotional, and mental sense of health and well being. This is what T'ai Chi is designed to promote.

Horary clock   Traditional Chinese Medicine's understanding of the ebb and flow of life energy patterns within the body. This understanding is used to treat various conditions using acupuncture, herbal, or QiGong therapy for optimum results.

Horse Stance   The basic stance for T'ai Chi, QiGong, and most martial arts.

Hypertension   High blood pressure caused most often by unmanaged stress. High blood pressure is the cause of most heart disease.

I-Ching   Also known as The Book of Changes; an ancient Chinese book of divination. The book is used to tell fortunes or to inspire people to look more deeply into themselves and their lives before making life decisions.

Jing Gong   *See* Sitting QiGong.

Kirlian photography   A photography method that appears to capture images of Qi or life energy.

Kuang Ping Yang style   The 64 movement long form of T'ai Chi brought to the West by master Kuo Lien Ying.

Lao-Tzu   The founder of Taoist philosophy.

Master   One who cultivates a clarity in life enabling them to be a nurturing force to themselves and the world.

Moving QiGong   Moving exercises, like T'ai Chi, that stimulate the flow of Qi through the body.

Mulan Quan style   A relatively modern form, yet rooted in a more ancient style. This may be the most elegant form of T'ai Chi, incorporating both dance and martial arts forms.

Post birth breathing   Normal abdominal T'ai Chi breathing.

Pre-birth breathing   A form of breathing that requires the abdominal muscles to draw in on an in breath, and relax out on an exhale.

Psychoneuroimmunology   The modern science of studying how the mind's attitudes and beliefs affect our physical health.

Push Hands   A sparring tool and/or a subtle tool for self awareness, whereby two partners (or opponents) engage in a dance like exchange becoming aware of one another's posture and balance. This can be carried to an extreme of pushing the opponent down when they are vulnerable, or merely becoming gently conscious of when they are vulnerable without actually pushing them down.

QiGong   "Breath work" or "energy exercise." There are about 7,000 QiGong exercises in the Chinese Medica (the bible of Chinese medicine).

Qi   Life energy. The Chinese character for Qi is also the character for air, as in breath.

Sensei   A teacher; a term of respect often used in martial arts circles.

Sifu   Chinese for one who has mastered an art. This term applies not only to martial arts as a master chef, or artist might be a sifu as well.

Sinking Qi   Settling the weight of the body into the leg you are shifting onto.

Sitting QiGong   Meditative exercises to promote the flow of Qi throughout the body.

333

Soong yi-dien   Loosen up. A T'ai Chi instruction to loosen the body, mind, and heart, encouraging the student to be more flexible and adaptable to all changes.

Spirit   The Latin root of "spirit" is "spir," to breathe, similar to the Chinese Qi, or life energy, expressed by the same word as "air."

Stress   In Traditional Chinese Medicine the result of unmanaged stress is blocked energy, and is the source of most physical, mental, emotional, and social problems.

T'ai Chi   A moving form of QiGong. Most Moving QiGong forms have only a few simple movements, and lack the continuous flow of the many multiple movements that T'ai Chi forms weave together.

T'ai Chi Ch'uan   "Supreme ultimate fist" or highest martial art.

Taoism   An ancient Chinese philosophy of life, which holds that the "Tao," the way of life, or the invisible force of nature's laws, can be accessed in states of alert calm. Regular immersion in the effortless power of life energy (through QiGong meditation) is believed to access the Tao for our lives, leading us to the most effortless and meaningful way to live.

Taoist Cannon   An ancient book that held all the early writing on QiGong, although at that time QiGong was called Tao-yin.

Taoist philosophy   Often thought of as T'ai Chi philosophy, because the subtle awareness of self and life energy, is so directly applicable to Taoism's goal of getting in touch with the Tao's natural laws and quiet power.

Tao-yin   Leading or guiding the energy, another ancient name for QiGong.

T-Cells   Cells that are believed to support our immune system by consuming virus, bacteria, and even tumor cells. T'ai Chi practice is believed to boost the body's production of T-Cells.

To gu na xin   Expelling the old energy, absorbing the new, which was another name for QiGong.

Traditional Chinese Medicine (TCM)   The Chinese health sciences that see the body and mind as a holistic entity united by the flow of life energy or Qi. The three main branches of TCM are acupuncture, herbal medicine, and exercises such as T'ai Chi and QiGong, often used in combination.

Vertical axis   The postural alignment for T'ai Chi.

Wan Yang-Ming   Philospher who fused the physical motions of T'ai Chi Ch'uan with the philosophy of Taoism.

Wu style   A formidable martial art form of T'ai Chi popular in many countries.

Yang Lu-Chan   The great grand master of Kuang Ping Yang Style, who created it after studying the Chen family style.

Yang style   A form of T'ai Chi very popular in the U.S. and China.

The Yellow Emperor's Classic of Chinese Medicine   The bible of Chinese Medicine in 200 BC. It stressed that "true medicine" is curing disease before it developes.

Yin & yang   The Chinese concepts of universal forces. All things are an eternally flowing interaction of two opposites; the ideal is healthy balance in all things. Yin is internal, dark, feminine, receptive. Yang is external, light, masculine, dynamic.

Zang-fu   In Chinese "solid-hollow." A system that indicates how Qi, life energy, flows throughout and between organs. It is the model of how the entire body is interlinked by that flow, and shows how treating associated organs or energy meridians can improve others.

Zazen   The Zen art of meditation. Directly translated it means "just sitting."

Zen   An oriental art of being here and now, allowing the mind and heart to let go of past and future attachments so that one can be fully immersed in the moment.

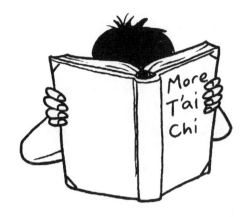

Living T'ai Chi's Effortless Power: Suggested Readings

Bach, Richard. *Jonathan Livingston Seagull*. New York: The Macmillan Company, 1970.

Badgley, M.D., Laurence. *Healing AIDS Naturally*. Foster City, CA: Human Energy Press, 1987.

Batmanghelidj, M.D., F. *The Body's Many Cries for Water*. Falls Church, VA: Global Health Solutions, Inc., 1997.

Behr, Ph.D., Thomas E. *The Tao of Sales*. Rockport, MA: Element Books, Inc., 1997.

Benson, M.D., Herbert. *The Relaxation Response*. New York: Avon Books, 1975.

Borysenko, Ph.D., Joan and Borysenko, Ph.D., Miroslav. *The Power of the Mind to Heal*. Carlsbad, CA: Hay House, Inc., 1994.

Capra, Fritjof (author of *the Tao of Physics*). *The Web of Life*. New York: Doubleday, 1996.

Chopra, Deepak. *Ageless Body, Timeless Mind*. New York: Harmony Books, 1993.

Cohen, Kenneth S. *The Way of QiGong: The Art and Science of Chinese Energy Healing*. New York: Ballantine Books, 1997.

Gerber, M.D., Richard. *Vibrational Medicine*. Santa Fe, New Mexico: Bear & Company, 1988.

Lee, Ph.D., Martin, with Emily, Melinda & Joyce Lee. *The Healing Art of T'ai Chi*. New York: Sterling Publishing Co. Inc., 1996.

Leight, Michelle Dominique. *The New Beauty, East-West Teachings in the beauty of body and soul*. New York: Kodansha America Inc., 1995.

Luk, Charles. *Taoist Yoga, Alchemy & Immortality*. York Beach, Maine: Samuel Weisner, Inc., 1973.

Mann, MB, LMCC, Felix. *Acupuncture, The Ancient Chinese Art of Healing*. New York: Random House, 1978.

Rothstein, Ed.D., Larry; Miller, Ph.D., Lyle H; and Smith, Ph.D., Alma Dell. *The Stress Solution*. New York: Pocket Books, a Division of Simon & Schuster, Inc., 1993.

Moyers, Bill. *Healing and the Mind*. New York: Doubleday, 1993.

Sandifer, Jon. *Acupressure for Health, Vitality and First Aid*. Rockport, MA: Element Books Limited, 1997.

Sang, Larry. *The Principles of Feng Shui*. Monterey Park, CA: The American Feng Shui Institute, 1994.

Talbot, Michael. *The Holographic Universe*. New York: HarperCollins Publishers, Inc., 1991.

Watts, Alan. *The Way of Zen*. New York: Vintage Books, A Division of Random House, Inc., 1985.

Weil, M.D., Andrew. *Spontaneous Healing*. New York: Ballantine Books, a Division of Random House, Inc., 1995.

Williams, Ph.D., Tom. *The Complete Illustrated Guide to Chinese Medicine*. Rockport, MA: Element Books, Inc., 1996.

Yutang, Lin. *The Wisdom of Laotse*. New York: The Modern Library, 1948.

Index

Enjoy a selection of fine T'ai Chi, QiGong, and Energy Work video and audio tapes and other stress management services, including T'ai Chi classes and *World T'ai Chi Getaway Vacations,* by Bill Douglas and Angela Wong-Douglas of Stress Management and Relaxation Technology (SMART).

SPECIAL RATE to readers of *The Complete Idiot's Guide to T'ai Chi & QiGong.*

Audios

QiGong Relaxation Therapy $12

A basic introduction to the wonders of relaxation therapy through energy work. This will open you up to the beautiful awareness of your body's flow of Qi, or life energy. This tape is used by some of the nations top corporations to help employees deal with stress. (Note: The Sitting QiGong exercise on this audio is also on the videos, *T'ai Chi; The Prescription for the Future,* Volume I *and T'ai Chi; The Ultimate Corporate Wellness Program.*)

QiGong for Children's Health and Relaxation $12

A fun-filled journey of self-awareness that you can practice yourself and pass on to your child or share the audio with your child flying through gentle adventures together. This tape is a great bedtime exercise (video *T'ai Chi for Kid's,* coming soon).

Expanding Awareness $12

This QiGong exercise connects you to the energy aspect of yourself and also to the field around you. A deep cleansing exercise to unload old stresses, enabling the body and field to fill with the perfection of Qi, or life energy.

An Earth Cleansing $12

This QiGong experience will help you touch into the healing aspects of the Earth. A centering tool that can ground your T'ai Chi practice in a very special way. The lying QiGong posture, or Floating on Earth Pose.

Videos

T'ai Chi & QiGong: The Prescription for the Future, Volume I $22.95
(Running time approx. 1 hour, 10 min.)

Introduces students to T'ai Chi philosophy, warm-up exercises, and beginning movements. Provides initial movements of the approximately 20-Minute Kuang Ping Yang Style's long form.

(Purchase this video plus Volumes II and III as a set for only $65.95)

T'ai Chi & QiGong: The Ultimate Corporate Wellness & Ergonomics Program $29.95
(Running time approx. 1 hour, 5 min.)

This introductory video explains to your employees T'ai Chi's wide-ranging benefits and how it works. The video culminates with a Sitting QiGong/Moving QiGong Relaxation Therapy and an introduction to initial T'ai Chi movements.

SMART also produces an ongoing series of 45-minute T'ai Chi/Stress Management Wellness Program class videos that can be purchased and used by your employees as an ongoing series for your own in-house Wellness Program. Or you can use this Wellness & Ergonomics video in conjunction with Volumes II and III below.

Video presenter and author, Bill Douglas, is available for corporate workshops and consultations to maximize the benefit of this unique program. He has been commissioned by companies such as Hallmark and Sprint corporations, Black & Veatch, and Associated Wholesale Grocers to teach employees and executive staffs these wonderful wellness tools. Visit Bill at his Web site: www.taichismart.com

T'ai Chi & QiGong: The Prescription for the Future, Volume II $22.95
(Running time approx. 1 hour, 5 min.)

This video takes students farther into the wonderful experience of Kuang Ping Yang Style's 20-minute long form, with more details on T'ai Chi movement to enrich your experience.

T'ai Chi & QiGong: The Prescription for the Future, Volume III $25.95 (Running time approx. 1 hour, 30 min.)

This video completes instruction of the nearly 20-minute Kuang Ping Yang long form. By teaching the most important aspect of T'ai Chi, the QiGong breathing method that accompanies each movement, Volume III brings students deep into the wonderful experience of T'ai Chi.

More of this *Prescription for the Future* series can be provided on request, enabling students to complete the entire Kuang Ping Yang Left Style as well.

Wheel Chair T'ai Chi; Kuang Ping Yang Style, Part I and *Children's T'ai Chi and QiGong Meditations* Videos COMING SOON!!!

Check SMART's World Wide Web page: www.taichismart.com for updates on new products, including health and mind expansion products and T'ai Chi fashion wear.

Mulan Quan Style T'ai Chi

Mulan Quan Basic Short Form & QiGong by Angela-Wong Douglas $27.95
(Running time approx. 1 hour, 30 min.)

This elegant form of T'ai Chi is perhaps one of the most delicately beautiful forms and is said to promote an elegant poised physique in practitioners. Although this video introduces the healing art of Moving QiGong, the Sitting QiGong on SMART's audio tape QiGong Relaxation Therapy is highly recommended as an adjunct to this Mulan video.

Mulan Quan Fan Style and Mulan Quan Sword Style instructional videos by Angela Wong-Douglas will soon be available as well, with moving QiGong warm ups. See SMART's Web page for details. The above Mulan Quan Basic video is a recommended prerequisite to the Fan and Sword Style videos.

T'ai Chi fans are available through SMART for $17.50. T'ai Chi retractable swords are $36. ($5 shipping for one sword.)

Add $4.50 shipping and handling for the first ordered item, and add $1.50 for each additional item. To order now, call 1-800-201-7892 (Ext. 14). Visa and Mastercard accepted.

Or order these and other SMART health and mind expansion products by visiting our Web Page at www.taichismart.com.

Or send your check or money order to:

Stress Management and Relaxation Technology
P.O. Box 7786
Shawnee Mission, KS 66207-0786

Allow 2 to 3 weeks for delivery.

If ordering by check or money order, complete the below form and enclose.

Ship to:

Name: _____

Address:_____

City/State/Zip: _____

Telephone: _____

E-mail: _____

Products ordered: _____Prices: _____

_____
_____
_____
_____
_____

On mail orders, Missouri residents add 6.6% sales tax.

Tax:_____
Shipping:_____
TOTAL:_____

Stress Management and Relaxation Technology (SMART) instructors can be contracted to conduct weekend seminars in any city (minimum enrollment required).

SMART also organizes *World T'ai Chi Getaways* to such places as Hawaii, China, Mexico, and other locations. For more information about these transformative holiday adventures, leave your name, address, and phone number to be added to the Getaway Mailing List by calling (913) 648-2256 or contact SMART through their Web page: www.taichismart.com

As trips are organized information will also be posted on SMART's World Wide Web page. Check SMART's World Wide Web Page regularly for updates on T'ai Chi health research, new health products, new services, and T'ai Chi accessories. This page is a great resource for everyone, *but especially health professionals, activities directors, and T'ai Chi instructors!*

www.taichismart.com is a touchstone for T'ai Chi, QiGong, and health care professionals around the world! The Web site offers the following:

- Comprehensive medical research on T'ai Chi and QiGong benefits.
- Updates on how T'ai Chi can be integrated into education, health care, business, court rehabilitation programs, etc.
- Information on "how to write for grants" for bringing T'ai Chi to society on all levels.
- Networking T'ai Chi groups from around the world to organize a "World T'ai Chi Day" to coincide with the UN's World Health Day.
- The best in T'ai Chi, QiGong, and health and mind expansion products and services.